Planning, Renovating, Expanding, and Constructing Library Facilities in Hospitals, Academic Medical Centers, and Health Organizations

Elizabeth Connor, MLS, AHIP
Editor

Routledge
Taylor & Francis Group
NEW YORK AND LONDON

First published in 2005 by Haworth press, Inc.
10 Alice Street, Binghamton, NY 13904-1580.

Published 2016 by Routledge
711 Third Avenue, New York, NY 10017, USA
2 Park Square, Milton Park, Abingdon, Oxon OX14 4RN

Routledge is an imprint of the Taylor & Francis Group, an informa business

The authors of Case Study 6 are employees of the U.S. Government. This work was prepared as part of their official duties. Title 17 U.S.C. 105 provides that "Copyright protection under this title is not available for any work of the United States Government." Title 17 U.S.C. 101 defines a United States Government work as a work prepared by a military service member or employee of the United States Government as part of that person's official duties. The views expressed in this article are those of the author(s) and do not reflect the official policy or position of the Department of the Navy, Department of Defense, or the United States Government.

Cover photos:
McIntyre Medical Sciences Building, McGill University, Montreal—Courtesy of Pamela J. Miller, Osler Library.

William H. Welch Medical Library, Johns Hopkins University—Courtesy of L. Gary Faulkner.

Health Sciences Learning Center, University of Wisconsin, Madison—Courtesy of Kahler/Slater, Architects.

Naval Medical Center, Portsmouth, Virginia—Official U.S. Navy photos.

Cover design by Kerry E. Mack.

Library of Congress Cataloging-in-Publication Data

Planning, renovating, expanding, and constructing library facilities in hospitals, academic medical centers, and health organizations / Elizabeth Connor, editor.
p. cm.
Includes bibliographical references and index.
ISBN-13: 978-0-7890-2540-1 (hc. : alk. paper)
ISBN-10: 0-7890-2540-X (hc. : alk. paper)
ISBN-13: 978-0-7890-2541-8 (pbk. : alk. paper)
ISBN-10: 0-7890-2541-8 (pbk. : alk. paper)
1. Medical libraries—United States—Case studies. 2. Hospital libraries—United States—Case studies. 3. Library buildings—United States—Design and construction—Case studies. 4. Library buildings—Remodeling—United States—Case studies.
[DNLM: 1. Libraries, Medical—organization & adminsitration. 2. Libraries, Hospital—organization & administration. 3. Facility Design and Construction. 4. Organizational Case Studies. Z 675.M4 P712 2005] I. Connor, Elizabeth, MLS.

Z675.M4P63 2005
026'.61—dc22

2005002619

ISBN 13: 978-0-78902-540-1 (hbk)

ABOUT THE EDITOR

Elizabeth Connor, MLS, AHIP, is Assistant Professor of Library Science and Science Liaison, The Citadel, Charleston, South Carolina, and is a distinguished member of the Academy of Health Information Professionals. She has extensive experience planning, designing, managing, and serving as consultant for library renovation and building projects at several institutions, and has a keen interest in ergonomics and collaborative workplaces. She is author of several peer-reviewed articles about medical informatics, electronic resources, search engines, and chat reference, and has written more than sixty book reviews for *Library Journal, Against the Grain, Bulletin of the Medical Library Association, Journal of the Medical Library Association, Medical Reference Services Quarterly,* and *The Post and Courier.* Ms. Connor is the author of the *Internet Guide to Travel Health,* the *Internet Guide to Food Safety and Security,* and editor of *A Guide to Developing End User Education Programs in Medical Libraries,* all published by The Haworth Press.

Planning, Renovating, Expanding, and Constructing Library Facilities in Hospitals, Academic Medical Centers, and Health Organizations

THE HAWORTH INFORMATION PRESS®
Medical Librarianship
M. Sandra Wood
Editor

A Guide to Developing End User Education Programs in Medical Libraries edited by Elizabeth Connor

Planning, Renovating, Expanding, and Constructing Library Facilities in Hospitals, Academic Medical Centers, and Health Organizations edited by Elizabeth Connor

Merrick Library in Merrick, New York,
created an inspirational and welcoming place
in a tiny, brown-shingled cottage,
and had the good sense to "hire" a resident cat.
Thank-you for giving me a library card
long before I learned to read.

CONTENTS

CONTRIBUTORS

Ralph D. Arcari, MLS, MA, PhD, is Associate Vice President for Academic Resources and Services; Director, Library; and Assistant Professor, Department of Community Medicine at the University of Connecticut Health Center, Farmington, Connecticut. Dr. Arcari teaches the history of medicine elective at the University of Connecticut School of Medicine.

Daniel Barkey, MBA, is Director, Information Technology at the University of Wisconsin–Madison.

Catherine M. Boss, MSLS, AHIP, is the Coordinator of Library Services at Jersey Shore University Medical Center in Neptune, New Jersey.

Willard F. Bryant Jr., MBA, is Associate Director, Finance and Administration at the William H. Welch Library of the Johns Hopkins University in Baltimore, Maryland.

Holly Shipp Buchanan, MLn, MBA, EdD, AHIP, is Associate Vice President for Knowledge Management and Information Technology, Director of the Health Sciences Library and Informatics Center, and Professor in the School of Medicine at the University of New Mexico Health Sciences Center, Albuquerque. She is the former Director of Libraries of the Medical College of Georgia in Augusta and prior to that was Director of Corporate Information Resources of the Alliant Health System in Louisville, Kentucky, and led library renovations at each of those institutions as well. Dr. Buchanan is a member of the Board of Regents of the National Library of Medicine and is past President of the Medical Library Association.

Jayne M. Campbell, MLS, is Associate Director, Information Services and Education at the William H. Welch Library of the Johns Hopkins University in Baltimore, Maryland.

Sylvia Contreras, MLIS, is Director of Oscar Rennebohm Library at Edgewood College in Madison, Wisconsin. She is the former Assistant Director for Library Operations at the Health Sciences Learning Center Library at the University of Wisconsin–Madison.

Stuart K. Dayton, MS, MFA, serves as Assistant Professor and Head of the Sievers Facility for Interactive Instruction and the Learning Resource Center at the McGoogan Library of Medicine at the University of Nebraska Medical Center. An accomplished artist, his graphic designs have won library marketing awards and are essential to communicating with the library's diverse constituencies.

Lisa R. Eblen, MLIS, is Health Sciences Library Division Officer at Naval Medical Center Portsmouth in Portsmouth, Virginia.

Tom Gensichen, MALS, established the Systems Department of the McGoogan Library of Medicine at the University of Nebraska Medical Center and has served as its Head since his appointment in 1990. Gensichen received his Master of Arts in Library Science from the University of Missouri, Columbia, and holds the earned rank of Associate Professor at the University of Nebraska Medical Center.

Mary E. Helms, MS, MA, AHIP, is Associate Professor and Associate Director, Library Resources and Technology at the McGoogan Library of Medicine, University of Nebraska Medical Center. Ms. Helms received her MS in Library and Information Science from Simmons College, Boston, and an MA in Management from Webster University, St. Louis. She teaches in the UNMC College of Medicine Integrated Clinical Experience curriculum and holds a courtesy appointment in the UNMC Department of Family Medicine.

Mary A. Hyde, MSLS, AHIP, has been director of the American College of Obstetricians and Gynecologists (ACOG) Resource Center for three years. She was also the reference librarian at the Resource Center during the most recent move. Before coming to the ACOG Resource Center, she started a library at the Association of American Medical Colleges.

Elisabeth Jacobsen, BA, has worked in medical library settings for over twenty-five years. She has a background in clinical librarianship and has designed and renovated several libraries. She has an undergraduate degree in English Literature from William Paterson University, Wayne, New Jersey, and has also studied Library and Information Science at Rutgers University. Ms. Jacobsen has been the Director of Library Services at Trinitas Hospital in Elizabeth, New Jersey, since 2000.

Deanna M. Lucia, MSLS, is the former Associate Director for Administrative Services at the University of Massachusetts Medical School's Lamar Soutter Library in Worcester.

Pamela J. Miller, BA, Academic Postgraduate Diploma in Archive Administration, is History of Medicine Librarian at the Osler Library of the History of Medicine, McGill University, Montreal. She is Montreal born and educated, having graduated with an Honours degree in Canadian History from McGill University. She received her professional education at University College, London, and worked as an archivist at the Hudson's Bay Company, London. She began work in the Osler Library after serving as Curator of Archival Collections at the McCord Museum of Canadian History. As History of Medicine Librarian, she supervised the Library's recent extensive renovations including the installation of climate control facilities. Her major interests are the history of medicine at McGill University, McGill's heritage collections, conservation, and exhibition.

Natalie Norcross, MLIS, MBA, is Assistant Director and Senior Academic Librarian at Ebling Library, University of Wisconsin–Madison. She began her professional career as head of Reference at the Chicago College of Osteopathic Medicine, and then was a hospital librarian in Hillsboro, Oregon, for many years, where she managed a clinical library and created a consumer health library. She also completed a National Library of Medicine fellowship in Medical Informatics and Outcomes Research at Oregon Health Sciences University. She is a distinguished member of the Academy of Health Information Professionals.

Kathleen Burr Oliver, MSLS, MPH, is Associate Director, Communications and Liaison Services at the William H. Welch Library of the Johns Hopkins University in Baltimore, Maryland.

Jane A. Pellegrino, MSLS, MALS, AHIP, is Library Services Department Head at Naval Medical Center Portsmouth in Portsmouth, Virginia.

Mary E. Piorun, MSLS, AHIP, is the Associate Director for Library Systems at the University of Massachusetts Medical School's Lamar Soutter Library in Worcester, and has been a member of the Academy of Health Information Professionals since 2000.

Marie Reidelbach, MLS, has held positions at the University of Nebraska Medical Center and the McGoogan Library of Medicine since 1981. She holds an MLS from Emporia State University in Emporia, Kansas, and was appointed Associate Director for User Services in 1998. Ms. Reidelbach holds the earned rank of Associate Professor as well as a courtesy appointment to the UNMC College of Nursing faculty.

Nancy K. Roderer, MLS, is Library Director of the William H. Welch Medical Library and Interim Director of the Division of Health Sciences Informatics of the Johns Hopkins University in Baltimore, Maryland.

Julie Schneider, MLS, is Head, Information Resources and Collection Development at the Ebling Library of the University of Wisconsin–Madison.

Erika Sevetson, MS, is Information Services Librarian at the Ebling Library of the University of Wisconsin–Madison.

Veronica Dawn Stewart, MLIS, is the Assistant Librarian at the Saint Francis Health Sciences Library of Saint Francis Health System in Tulsa, Oklahoma.

Janis Teal, MLS, MAT, AHIP, is Deputy Director for Library Services at the University of New Mexico Health Sciences Library and Informatics Center, Albuquerque. During her ten years at the library, there have been continuous remodeling projects. She is the former Director of the Hupp Medical Library, Ohio Valley Medical Center, Wheeling, West Virginia, where she participated in the design and construction of a new library within the hospital.

Pamela Van Hine, MSLS, AHIP, was director of the American College of Obstetricians and Gynecologists (ACOG) Resource Center for more than twenty years before stepping down to a part-time position in 2002. While she was director, she moved the Resource Center three times.

Nancy N. Woelfl, PhD, serves as Director of McGoogan Library of Medicine at the University of Nebraska Medical Center, a position she has held since 1987. Ms. Woelfl received her MLS and a doctorate in library and information science from Case Western Reserve University in Cleveland, Ohio. She is a career health sciences librarian and prior to appointment at the University of Nebraska Medical Center, held positions at the Ohio State and Case Western Reserve University health sciences libraries, as well as at the NASA Lewis Research Center in Cleveland. Dr. Woelfl holds the rank of Professor and in addition to her work in the library, studies the effect of learning style on problem-based learning in medicine.

T. Elizabeth Workman, MLIS, is an Associate Librarian at the Spencer S. Eccles Health Sciences Library, and also manages the Hope Fox Eccles Clinical Library in University Hospital. She received her library degree from the University of Hawai'i at Manoa.

Foreword

As of late, much library literature focuses on discussions of the changing nature of library services and spaces. Declining gate counts, the rise of Internet search engines, the increasing amount of freely available information on the Web, and changes in student study habits are distinctive trends that cause many to question the future of the librarian's traditional role as organizer and provider of information resources, and indeed, the need for physical space for the library itself. Articles describing "deserted libraries" where gate counts and circulation are falling as students find new study spaces in dorm rooms or apartments, coffee shops, or nearby bookstores, have led administrators to question why they should support library construction or renovation, especially when students, faculty, and the general public now tend to look to the Internet for answers rather than the library. In this environment, funding and designing new buildings are particularly challenging.

However, the collected descriptions of libraries that follow paint a much more positive picture about the futures of librarians and the futures of libraries. These case studies depict librarians who have taken on a wide variety of new roles, from informationists and educators to archivists and knowledge managers. They describe libraries that have filled empty spaces left by shrinking their print collections with new services ranging from classroom spaces, to visualization laboratories, to consumer health collections. They highlight expanded roles for libraries as places where all members of the community can come together, as repurposed and expanded learning centers, and as places for intellectual pursuits. Their planning processes point also to vast amounts of printed material that still must be preserved and organized; they question the ability of the Web to deliver quality information; and they look askance at the disorganized nature of information on the Internet.

An examination of these case studies shed additional light on the physical nature of the future library and emerging space-related themes. Through them, evidence is provided that libraries will continue to provide group study spaces for individuals to engage in quiet pursuits, and spaces to provide training in the use of information resources. Users will demand spaces that are comfortable for thinking and working, conducive to long periods of screen use, and that have support systems and help in place as well as quality output devices such as printers or high-definition screens. Browsing will be an essential function of libraries, and libraries will retain a symbolic significance for scholars. The library will also continue to be important as a repository of older physical information sources, although this information may be stored only in a few low-cost repositories. Infrastructure, amenities, and "presence" will characterize our libraries; high-tech facilities such as electronic classrooms, information arcades, faculty support centers, and library cafés will be omnipresent; and portable computing will become ubiquitous. Libraries will have computer-equipped classrooms and ample access to public computing facilities, and library buildings will continue to provide places for people and their activities rather than materials storage.

Health sciences libraries such as those described in this text have been redesigning their facilities to meet the needs of not only the current generation of users but also the needs of the next generation of scholars, scientists, and clinicians who will have the information-seeking skills, not to mention the patience needed to locate quality information. Their libraries provide a mix of group and individual study spaces, combined service points that assist users with both technology and the use of information resources, and place more emphasis on consumer health information, and more attractive spaces. These facilities reflect the impact that environmental changes in scholarly communication, technology, and preferred learning environments are having on current library building design. They also demonstrate the importance of remembering several important rules about building for change:

1. Spaces that work well over time are spaces that are built around very fundamental human needs such as comfort, natural light, and good social ambience.

2. Rigidity of building space around particular technologies is to be avoided.
3. Technology will become more sophisticated, less obtrusive, and less visible.
4. The engagement of technology with culture is unpredictable.

Finally, the designers and managers of these library facilities have remembered that what a library is depends on what a library does.

Logan Ludwig, PhD, AHIP
Library Buildings Consultant and Buildings Editor,
Journal of the Medical Library Association;
Associate Dean, Library and Telehealth Services,
Loyola University Health System,
Maywood, Illinois

Introduction

Today's library users expect comfortable and inviting spaces to consult, connect, collaborate, focus, learn, teach, and reflect. Few library buildings provide the accessibility, functionality, or flexibility needed over the long term to support collections, services, technology, and people in new and expansive ways. The challenge of renovating an existing library, constructing an addition, or building a new library requires an enormous amount of organizational skill, resourcefulness, creativity, stamina, and willingness to compromise. Librarians often seek knowledge of best practices and innovative approaches to improve the quality of services offered by their institutions. This book contains descriptive and practical information for hospital, academic health sciences, health association, and other special librarians who are planning to refurbish, renovate, or construct a library in the near or distant future, and for students interested in learning more about this subject.

In October and November 2003, several calls for contributions were sent to MEDLIB-L Listserv, which is devoted to medical librarianship, several regional mailing lists, and persons known to have worked with science, technology, and medical library building projects. These announcements asked librarians who have renovated or built a library in the last three to five years to consider submitting a case study for a forthcoming book about library buildings. Interested librarians were asked to submit a structured abstract that described setting, objectives, methods, results, and conclusions. Librarians selected to participate were sent detailed style instructions and expected to submit first drafts by February 2004.

The case studies featured here represent the ideas, experiences, and approaches of thirteen private and public institutions in the United States and Canada, with contributed case studies from librarians working in associations, health care systems, teaching hospitals, medical schools, and academic medical centers in Connecticut, Maryland, Massachusetts, Nebraska, New Jersey, New Mexico, Oklahoma, Utah, Virginia, Washington, DC, Wisconsin, and Montreal, Canada.

The thirteen case studies range from designing, refurbishing, renovating, and refurnishing existing library space; merging library collections, services, and staffs; and constructing multimillion-dollar library buildings. The cases in this book follow a format similar to the structured abstract, including setting, objectives, methods, results, and conclusions. Some case studies are illustrated and may be supplemented by additional documents. Space does not allow inclusion of every diagram, photograph, or illustration related to the projects. Readers are welcome to explore the Web sites featured in this work to find more detailed information about specific libraries, and to contact librarians whose projects interest or intrigue them.

Themes common to the case studies include the importance of involving library faculty/staff in the planning processes; engaging the services of a library consultant; visiting other libraries and buildings to get ideas; keeping library patrons aware of project progress; understanding the language and tools used by architects, engineers, and designers; reviewing plans and project progress on a regular basis, including frequent walk-throughs of the construction site; and acknowledging and celebrating people for their professional expertise and contributions of time and energy.

These ideas, insights, and approaches can be used, adapted, or expanded by others. Learn from these experiences to improve or develop a physical facility that supports your institution's goals and objectives.

Elizabeth Connor, MLS, AHIP
Charleston, South Carolina

PART I: SPECIAL LIBRARIES

Case Study 1

ACOG Resource Center Happily Moves to the Basement

Mary A. Hyde
Pamela Van Hine

OVERVIEW

Setting: The American College of Obstetricians and Gynecologists (ACOG) is the national professional association for more than 40,000 obstetrician-gynecologists. The ACOG Resource Center includes the J. Bay Jacobs Library, a collection on the history of American obstetrics and gynecology. The Resource Center is used on-site by staff, committee members, and historians. Although the Resource Center handles more than 100,000 requests per year, most are not received from on-site visitors. The library had outgrown its space, and the existing space was needed for the college journal's editorial office, which was being moved in-house. The librarians agreed to move into the basement, gaining twice as much space.

Objective: The overall planning objective was to turn an awkwardly shaped basement space into a warm, welcoming space that enticed users, met the needs of library staff, comfortably

The authors would like to thank the following current and former ACOG staff: Mary Hay Glass for her background research, negotiations, and her input in planning of the new library; Debra Scarborough for her photograph of the History Library and the fact-checking she did on the History Library; Mimi Nugent, Pat Rockinberg, and Margaret Goodman for their input on the budget and the HVAC systems and project coordination; Marian Wiseman for the photographs from *ACOG Today*; and Elsa Brown and Dr. Ralph Hale for their advocacy and unwavering support of the project.

housed the collections for many years, provided sufficient space and wiring for technology, and provided four separate environmentally controlled zones—from "the refrigerator," for the oldest and rarest books and archives, to the general reading area, with plenty of light and relative warmth.

Methods: In 2000, the librarians developed surveys for library users and staff, visited recently renovated or new libraries, and refreshed their knowledge about space planning. The planning document included a summary of fifteen prioritized needs for the new space. Building staff selected the architect and prepared the budget. In June 2000, staff presented their needs to the architects. Construction started in July and was completed by winter. The library was moved in mid-December 2000.

Results/conclusions: The overall new space is efficient, functional, and well-designed, meets most of the space requirements, and is a beautiful and welcoming showcase for the college. With careful planning and groundwork, it is possible to create a wonderful library, even in the basement.

INTRODUCTION

The purpose of this chapter is to describe the decision-making and developmental processes involved in designing and building the new space for the Resource Center, the library of The American College of Obstetricians and Gynecologists (ACOG), in Washington, DC.

Setting

The ACOG is the national professional association for more than 40,000 obstetrician-gynecologists. The ACOG Resource Center, the college library, serves ACOG staff, committees, officers, and members. Resource Center staff also serve nonmembers, primarily by providing them with materials produced by ACOG. On-site use represents a small part of the more than 100,000 requests/year handled by the Resource Center. Most requests come through e-mail, facsimile, telephone, or mail. On-site users are primarily college staff, committee members, historians, and visitors.

The Resource Center also includes the J. Bay Jacobs Library, a special collection on the history of American obstetrics and gynecology that was started in 1983 and has its own staff, programs, activities, and special environmental needs. A specific fund-raising project for the History Library established a self-sustaining endowment for the ongoing support of the library. The History Library is a source of pride for ACOG members and an impressive focal point of ACOG tours.

The Resource Center, which was started in 1969 with a room filled with miscellaneous books and journals, expanded and moved several times before the current expansion. Major moves and expansions coincided with moves of the college—from Chicago to Washington, DC, in 1981; and from 6th and Maryland SW to a new building at 12th and DSW in Washington, DC, in 1988. Librarians acquired additional shelf space in other parts of ACOG as the shelf space in the library became full, and some of this additional space was lost when it was needed for other purposes. By 1995, the Resource Center and History Library had outgrown their available shelf space (see Table 1.1).

Because of the library's prime location—on the same floor with the primary college meeting rooms and reception area—the library could not expand further in its current location. Approximately 200

TABLE 1.1. Growth of collection and services.

Year	Shelving used	Available shelving	FTE library staff	Requests
1979	267.0	267	5	26,400
1981	330.0	337	5	34,000
1983	434.0	710	5	38,000
1985	736.0	797	5.5	62,000
1987	863.0	895	7.5	77,000
1989	944.0	1,160	9.5	97,000
1992	1,088.7	1,332	11.5	97,000
1994	1,211.0	1,320	5.5	100,000+
2000	1,690.7[a]	1,445.2	6	100,000+

Source: Pamela Van Hine.
[a]Includes off-site storage.

linear feet of shelf space was made available in a basement storage room, but was filled by 1996. In 1997, the History Library received the Burnhill Collection, a very large donation that required off-site storage arrangements. Although the librarians continued to use off-site storage to contain the overflow of library materials, by 1999 they needed a better and larger space in-house. Serendipitously, the existing library staff space was needed for the college journal's editorial office, which was moving in-house. When the library director was asked if library staff would be willing to move into the basement, gaining twice as much space, she agreed.

Objective

The overall objective of library staff was to turn an awkwardly shaped basement into a warm, welcoming space that enticed library users. The new space had to meet the needs of library staff, comfortably house the collections for many years, provide sufficient space and wiring for technology, and provide four separate environmentally controlled zones—from "the refrigerator," for the oldest and rarest books and archives, to the general reading area, with plenty of light and relative warmth. The planning period—from start to finish—was less than one year. The librarians received confirmation in January 2000 that they needed to move by the end of the year.

METHODS

The goals of library space planning were to identify what currently worked well, what needed to be done differently, what no longer needed to be done, what new work was to be performed, which spaces were needed to accomplish all of the library functions, and how these spaces were to be integrated. In planning their new library space, Resource Center librarians were fortunate in many ways. The library director and office management staff had collaboratively planned the two prior library spaces. The director was in the middle of her house renovation, which gave her hands-on experience working with architects, builders, and blueprints. Library staff worked with a supportive administration, a generous budget, and architects who listened to them and understood their needs. Finally, the library is located in a major metropolitan area with ready access to many libraries, librarians, and experts in all areas of library space planning.

Methods used by library staff to help plan the library included developing staff and patron surveys; analyzing trends in space needs, staffing, and use; reviewing prior planning records; searching for and reviewing information on library planning;[1] visiting other recently renovated or new libraries; getting bids and reviews for specific projects; identifying a library planning consultant for the project; and coordinating the project through many meetings.

Staff Survey

The librarians developed a survey for library staff to determine which workspace features should be kept, what needed to be changed, and what ideal workspaces would be. Librarians also hoped that the questionnaire would help engage library staff in the planning process, help them feel that their views mattered, and get them excited about the new space. The open-ended questions covered five other topics, in addition to workspace: the general library space and functions, proposed workroom, collection arrangement, equipment, and their vision for the new library. Library staff were also encouraged to be involved in many planning meetings and on specific planning projects. Their input was sought for specific issues that affected their work.

User Survey

The librarians also developed a survey for library patrons to gather their suggestions on what current library features should be kept, which should be changed, and what new features were needed. The questionnaire was one way to engage patrons in library planning and get them excited about the new space. The two-page questionnaire covered six topics: user areas, equipment, collection arrangement, general library functional spaces, general questions (e.g., best and worst current features, most needed new feature), and their vision for future library space and services. After staff review, the final version was sent electronically to about fifty key library users. Only ACOG staff were surveyed as they are the only group that routinely uses the library in-house. Patrons could complete the form electronically or print it out and write their responses on the printed copy. Printed copies were also available in the library. Initial nonresponders were sent a follow-up request. Forty completed questionnaires, representing forty-four patrons, were returned—providing an excellent mix of responses from primary library patrons at all levels.

Library Visits

In the first half of 2000, Resource Center librarians visited several recently renovated or new libraries. Libraries of all types and sizes included new public, academic, federal, and special libraries in San Francisco, California; New York City; Seattle, Washington; Portland, Oregon; Vancouver, British Columbia, Canada; Washington, DC; Hanover, New Hampshire; Burlington, Vermont; and Alexandria, Virginia. Visits were arranged in conjunction with other business in the area to keep costs down. The librarians developed a brief list of open-ended questions to ask the host librarians and toured as much of each library as possible. The questions focused on what the librarians liked and did not like about the new library and what they would have done differently.

Space Planning Consultant

A library space planning consultant is essential for a librarian who has never planned a new library, and helpful for librarians with previous library planning experience. The consultant should be more current on library planning issues (e.g., planning for evolving technologies) than the typical librarian. Also, the consultant can confirm the librarian's plans and planning process, and, most important, the consultant can serve as the librarian's advocate in the planning process—an outside authority who can champion the needs of the librarian in an unbiased way. For these reasons, Resource Center librarians wanted to identify a library space planning consultant to work with them.

Several potential consultants were identified through Special Libraries Association (SLA), Medical Library Association (MLA), and Regional Medical Library (RML) resources, and references were checked for the most promising candidates. Before meeting with their first choice, the librarians carefully determined what they wanted the consultant to provide and prepared questions, including exactly how the consultant bills for services and approximately what those services will cost.

Library Movers

Unless the collection is very tiny, use professional movers to move the library to its new location. The movers should be experienced in moving libraries because organizing and preparing library materials takes special knowledge for a successful and efficient move. Use all possible resources to identify candidates: national and local library associations, mailing lists, and RML resources, then ask for references and contact some of them to find out if they were satisfied with the work. Librarians should meet with the final choices—to ensure compatibility, review the work needed, go over the process, ask for suggestions, and request formal bids.

RESULTS

Staff Survey

All seven library staff completed the survey, although some provided more comprehensive information than others. The results were not as useful as the authors hoped they would be, but certain issues were frequently raised. Staff clearly needed more storage space, convenient access to work supplies, a workroom, and a bigger reference desk. Staff needed access to a typewriter, a larger copier, and a facsimile machine, but not in their immediate work areas. They also supported enhanced patron areas that were separate from the reference desk and their work areas. Staff were happy with current file cabinets, shelving with the pullout shelves, although they agreed that many more of both were needed. Poor environmental control was also cited as a problem, especially in the History Library.

User Survey

Forty-four library patrons completed forty questionnaires (88 percent return rate), although not everyone answered every question. The users were supportive of the new library and provided many excellent suggestions for the new space. Patrons wanted three different types of user areas: a large library table so they could spread out their work, more public access computer stations on carrels that had room for books, and a pleasant and comfortable reading area for more casual work. They wanted better lighting and signage; a larger, better copier and a place to store books and journals while making copies; and to be able to get copies of ACOG publications without disturbing library staff. Patrons did not want to climb on a stepstool to take materials off upper shelves. Most of them did not know what compact shelving was, but they thought it was satisfactory for older, less frequently used materials. Some of the most useful responses were about their vision for the new library and future library services. Patrons described the new library as spacious, open, welcoming, inviting, appealing, attractive, well-lit, easy to use, and user-friendly. The new space would have plants, coffee, computers, and knowledgeable staff who provide relevant and timely information.

Library Visits

Visiting other libraries was invaluable to Resource Center librarians, who saw brilliant designs as well as puzzling ones. Host librarians were honest in their appraisals of the new space and suggested innovative and creative solutions that may not have occurred to the authors. Lessons learned covered efficiency, functionality, flexibility, beauty, planning processes, and miscellaneous tips.

In the efficient library, the layout of the space and location of equipment and furniture matches the workflow of library staff and habits of library users, which requires that the librarians fully understand how both groups use the existing space before planning the new library. Tips include fitting shelving into the rectangular areas to maximize shelf space and to use oddly shaped spaces for other functions. Furnishing should fit the space efficiently.

The functional library provides space and furnishings that enable library staff and patrons to work easily and productively. Furniture can serve several functions. For example, the tops of low, flat storage cabinets can also be used as work areas. Planning for shelving and lighting is a key functionality issue. The walls and floors should support the shelving, and attention must be paid to shelf and ceiling heights. Different functions require different types of lighting. Ceiling lights need to be laid out carefully, with consideration of the location of shelving and furniture. Retrofitting shelving or lighting can be very expensive, if it is possible at all.

The flexible library provides staff and user areas that are adaptable to meet future needs. Although cubicle staff workspaces are the easiest to change, they may not provide sufficient privacy for some library staff. The solution in one library was to use moveable walls for staff offices. The flexible library also provides a variety of seating and work areas for library patrons, including computer stations. Study carrels should be adjustable to hold different combinations of equipment, library materials, and users. "Wired" library tables may be more flexible than traditional study carrels.

The well-planned library is also beautiful, but not at the expense of efficiency, functionality, or flexibility. Consulting a library space planner may be useful to achieve the right balance between beauty and library function.

The well-designed library has a carefully developed planning process. As soon as possible, set up a committee of key players and decision makers, including library staff, library patrons, and administration. Architects, builders, and a library space planning consultant can be included after the initial meetings. Set up subgroups to work on specific tasks, meet regularly, and keep everyone informed and involved. Everyone should feel that his or her needs are being met. Finally, remember to say thanks to everyone who helped.

Other tips gleaned from visits addressed promotion, branding, signage, color, protecting surfaces, and unusual collaborations. To encourage use of the new library, plan to promote the new library through an open house, tours, orientation sessions, newsletters, and intranet/Internet announcements. Find creative ways and designs to indicate the "brand" of the parent organization and library through signage, plaques, rugs, art work, displays, etched letters in doors, wall maps, and handouts. All signage should be attractive, clear, well-designed, and easily changeable. Information should be provided in multiple formats—wall maps, handouts, and specific area signage. Use color effectively, as it is a key part of a well-designed library. Protect the work surfaces of furnishings that will have hard use such as the reference desk and photocopying area. Use sturdy and easy-to-clean materials and use colors that will not show dirt. Finally, when the opportunity arises, do something a little different. Make room for coffee, a bookstore, a museum, and a learning lab; integrate the library with other services such as a store, cafeteria, or gymnasium.

Space Planning Consultant

The authors identified an excellent, experienced library space planning consultant, checked her references, and met with her to determine objectives, process, costs, and compatibility. However, her services were not used because the planning process for the library went so well. If the consultant had been used, we would have requested a formal proposal from her.

Meetings with Various Experts

Meetings included discussing broad-based issues with administration; putting together a list of priorities for the new library; meeting initially with the architects; and meeting later to discuss the blueprints and make any final changes to the plans. The librarians met with administration on several occasions to agree upon the planning process and budget, and to discuss the needs and roles of various individuals involved in planning the new library. They had the opportunity to explain the basic philosophy of their library services, why the collection would continue to have books and journals, and why everything is not on the Internet. Librarians prepared background documents to support their viewpoints and found that the Dartmouth Library planning documents were extremely helpful for this effort.[2]

After reviewing their survey results and the results of visiting other libraries, the librarians developed a prioritized list of fifteen goals for the new library space (see Appendix A). The most important consideration was having more shelf space—at least twice the current space. Fortunately, because the new library would be in the basement, the structure could support compact shelving, which was the only way to provide that much shelving in the available space. Request more shelf space than needed, because even with adjustable shelves, some shelf space is often not useable, as medical books and journals are often taller than typical library materials (see Table 1.2).

The librarians met with the architects and office management staff in June, gave them their prioritized list, survey results, and other background materials, and discussed their needs. Office management staff presented their needs, including the need to reuse existing library shelving and furnishings when possible. The architects listened carefully and presented several terrific ideas. Office staff prepared the final budget (see Appendix B).

By July, the architects provided a final blueprint that was a brilliant design that met most of the needs on the librarians' wish list. The librarians made a few minor changes to the plans to create a space for the history fellow, expand staff workspace, and install a small coat closet. The design provided a combination of compact and regular shelving that met shelving space needs and reused most of the existing shelving (see Photo 1.1).

TABLE 1.2. Comparison of old and new library space.

	Square-feet floor space	Linear shelf feet
Old library	2,025	1,445.2[a]
New library	3,800	4,295[b]

Source: Pamela Van Hine.
[a]On-site only (1,690.7 if including off-site storage).
[b]Theoretical (~3,500 functional linear shelf feet in new space).

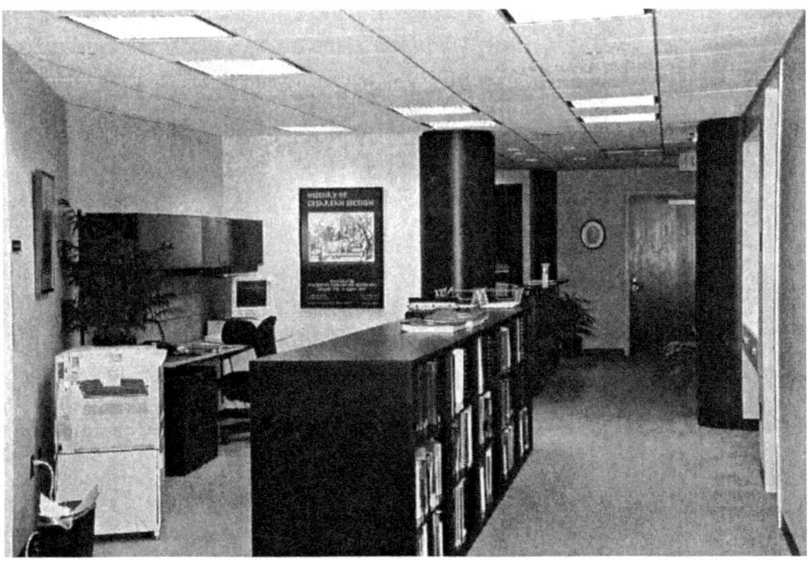

PHOTO 1.1. Reference collection and workstation for history fellow. Photograph by Marian Wiseman; first published in "New Digs for Resource Center and History Library." *ACOG Today* 45(9): 15, October 2001, © The American College of Obstetricians and Gynecologists. Used with permission.

The design provided a dramatic and impressive entrance through double glass doors, mimicking the reception area on the main floor. The new reference desk is more than twice as large as the old one and has ample room for two people (see Photo 1.2).

The desk is surrounded by some of the History Library shelving. The History Library has two separate environmental zones but has been incorporated into the overall library. It is attractive and inviting, with its etched glass door and lovely curved bookcases. Visitors can choose from a variety of seating—four computer stations (one with scanner), two comfortable chairs under the window, or a long table that seats six to eight persons (or one editor with many books). One entire long wall is filled with floor-to-ceiling file cabinets and storage cabinets, with convenient access by library staff who work across from them. Space was found for a small workroom for library staff. But most important, a horridly cramped and uninviting space was opened up to create a lovely and welcoming library that is a source of pride and a showcase for the college (see Photos 1.3 and 1.4).

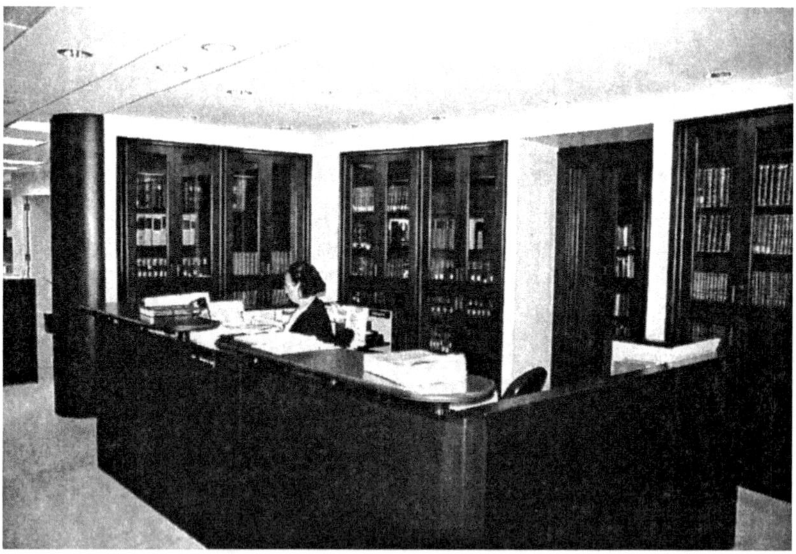

PHOTO 1.2. Reference desk. Photograph by Marian Wiseman; first published in "New Digs for Resource Center and History Library." *ACOG Today* 45(9): 15, October 2001, © The American College of Obstetricians and Gynecologists. Used with permission.

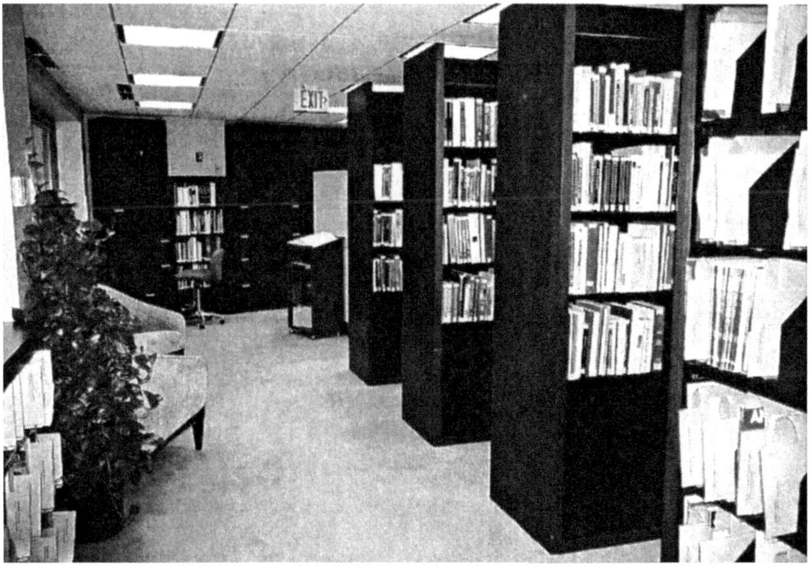

PHOTO 1.3. Reading room, lounge seating, and windows. Photograph by Marian Wiseman; first published in "New Digs for Resource Center and History Library." *ACOG Today* 45(9): 15, October 2001, © The American College of Obstetricians and Gynecologists. Used with permission.

MOVING THE COLLECTION

The librarians identified potential movers through SLA, MLA, and RML sources and checked references for the three final choices. They met with representatives from the three finalists, discussed their moving needs and how the vendor would handle the move, and requested formal bids from the finalists. Fortuitously, the least-expensive bidder also gave the best, most carefully thought out presentation, and was the most compatible with library staff.

Moving the Resource Center required interweaving materials from several locations, as well as leaving space for new materials. The librarians carefully measured existing collections, laid out where different materials would go in the new library, calculated space needed for short-term growth, and prepared lists and signs indicating exactly how much shelf space to allot for each section or journal title and which shelves to use in the new library. The library had to be moved in one

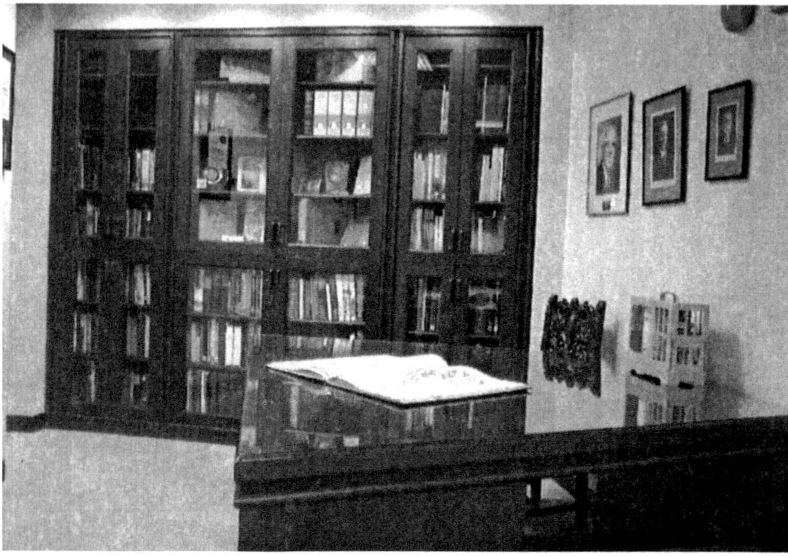

PHOTO 1.4. History Library. Photograph by Debra G. Scarborough. Used with permission.

day, so three librarians worked with four teams of movers simultaneously—moving the History Library from one location to its new shelving, and moving the Resource Center from one location to its new shelving. In retrospect, the librarians regret that they did not have the opportunity to measure the shelf heights or mark specific locations on the new shelving before moving day. Some shelves had to be adjusted or removed before shelving the collection, wasting precious time.

After the Move

Even a well-planned move will not go perfectly. After the move, determine what is not working correctly and arrange to get it fixed. Keep a punch list of problems and periodically check that they are being resolved. Once you have moved in, encourage your patrons to use the new library. Order and install signs, provide instruction sheets, hang pictures, "brand" the space with institution-specific banners and plaques, offer tours, send out announcements, and have a welcome party. Consider a follow-up questionnaire for library staff and patrons to see if the new space meets their expectations and to see what enhancements should be considered.

RECOMMENDATIONS

Based on experience planning and implementing this project for the ACOG Resource Center, the authors offer the following recommendations to others planning similar projects:

- Understand the role of the library in your institution and how the new library can enhance that role.
- Read about library space planning and research your specific needs.
- Gain the support and involvement of all library staff; make sure that their needs are met.
- Get suggestions and support from your primary library users; get them involved and excited.
- Work with your administration to get the best new library possible.
- Dream big, know exactly what you want, prioritize your needs, and be willing to make compromises.
- Visit as many new or remodeled libraries as you can; get design ideas and tips; ask the library staff what they like and what they would have done differently.
- Identify a reputable library planning consultant to work with you and support you; meet with the consultant to discuss your needs and to ensure your compatibility; work with the consultant as needed.
- For each planning project, get multiple bids from reputable sources and evaluate them according to your institution's guidelines. Always get a list of prior clients and contact some of them to get a sense of overall client satisfaction.
- Set up a good project tracking system. Keep detailed, organized plans and schedules.
- Understand your architects, blueprints, and the building process.
- Ensure that your architects understand your needs and priorities; prior experience building libraries is highly desirable.
- Ensure that everyone knows who is responsible for which projects.
- Meet your deadlines, and keep changes minimal to keep costs down.

- Schedule frequent meetings. Stay informed and keep everyone else informed.
- Monitor work in progress to ensure that everything is installed according to the blueprints.
- Take your own before and after pictures.
- Follow up after the move.

CONCLUSION

The overall new space for the ACOG Resource Center is efficient, functional, and well-designed, meets most space requirements, and is a beautiful and welcoming showcase for the college. With careful planning and groundwork, it is possible to create a wonderful library, even in the basement.

APPENDIX A: SPACE PRIORITIES AND GOALS

Rank	Space planning goals	Achieved
1	Develop maximum shelf space in Resource Center/History Library—at least 3,000 feet. Shelving can include compact shelving.	New library has 4,295 feet of shelving (~3,500 functional feet).
2	Provide good environmental control throughout library for temperature, humidity, lighting, airflow, and air quality. Environment should be constant, within guidelines, and healthy for books and people.	New space has four separate environmental zones.
3	Provide better lighting throughout, including specific task lighting.	Lighting is much better than in old library, but some task lighting is still needed and some compact shelving areas are too dark.
4	Prepare signage throughout.	Signage is still needed.
5	Provide a variety of types of spaces for users: carrels, library tables, and lounge area. No user area should be immediately next to the reference desk.	The new library has three different types of user spaces that are sufficient for current needs.
6	Build a much larger reference desk.	The new one is more than twice as large and deep as the old one.

Rank	Space planning goals	Achieved
7	Incorporate a multipurpose workroom that includes storage space (to replace three storage closets in old library).	Space was found for a small, compact workroom. It is not large enough for all of the planned functions, but other workspaces help compensate.
8	Provide more public-access computers and wiring for personal computers.	New library has four public-access computers and wiring for personal computers in several places.
9	Provide more file cabinets.	Some additional file space was provided, especially near workspaces. Storage units were fit on top of the file cabinets to provide additional storage space. More cabinets will be needed.
10	Enhance staff space by providing more space, more ergonomic desks, better lighting, more file space, and a better layout.	The new staff spaces are well-designed and efficient, but not ergonomically correct for keyboarding. Ergonomic keyboard holders will need to be added.
11	Provide places to view audiovisuals/multimedia.	No specific space was designated for this function, but the history fellow space can be used for personal viewing and CD-ROMs can be run from several library computers.
12	Provide better space for training on library computers.	The public-access computers have sufficient space for small group training or detailed one-on-one training. Other ACOG facilities can be used for larger classes.
13	Incorporate an office space for history fellow, space for library interns, and space for future staff growth.	The architects created an open desk area for the history fellow. The staff cubicles have a designated desk for an intern and sufficient space to add staff.
14	Include more than one copier and offer better copier features in a noise-controlled area that is close to the journals. Library staff should have easy access to the second copier.	The new library has one copier that is close to the journals and has a place to store materials to be copied. Library staff no longer have a copier immediately next to them, but they have access to two large copiers in a room beyond the library.

Rank	Space planning goals	Achieved
15	Miscellaneous needs include coat closet, new book display area, new journal display area, space for book carts, materials to be shelved, space for ACOG pamphlets and other books, library bulletin board, visitor phone, and storage space for audiovisuals.	The architects were not able to create a space for new books or journals without cutting overall shelf space. Other needs were met, although a bulletin board—or equivalent—is still needed.

APPENDIX B: BUDGET SUMMARY FOR NEW ACOG RESOURCE CENTER, 2000

Item	Estimate	Final bid	Final cost
Compact shelving	$109,800	$109,800	$115,923.75
Carpeting	26,000	26,000	29,896.80
HVAC and mechanical systems	100,000	—	58,932.00
Electrical and lighting	70,000	61,000	59,457.00
Telephone and cabling	3,500	—	4,675.30
Ceiling	13,000	—	12,600.00
Electronic security	3,500	—	3,700.00
Plumbing	1,200	—	1,350.00
Sprinkler/fire alarm	16,000	—	9,484.68
Millwork (reworking existing shelving)	—	83,000	67,467.00
Furniture, file cabinets	10,000	—	73,208.21
Drywall finish, painting, demolition, construction	5,000	—	36,909.98
Design, blueprints	—	20,000	17,670.00
Consultants for mechanicals	10,000	—	1,440.00
Moving library—collection and furnishings	3,000 (collection only)	—	24,692.00
Total			$517,406.72

NOTES

1. Cohen, A. and Cohen, E. *Designing and Space Planning for Libraries: A Behavioral Guide.* New York: Bowker, 1979.

2. *Report of the Task Force on the Library of the 21st Century: The Berry and Baker Libraries.* Available online at: <http://www.dartmouth.edu/~library/Berry Baker/task.html>.

Case Study 2

Preserving Medical History: Recent Renovations to the Osler Library

Pamela J. Miller

OVERVIEW

Setting: The Osler Library was established in 1919 from Sir William Osler's bequest of his collection of 8,000 rare books on the history of medicine and science. Concentrating on the history and social studies of medicine, the library currently holds 22,000 rare books, 33,000 circulating books, 300 meters of archives, and about 600 artifacts. The Osler Library of the History of Medicine at McGill University is located in a round, fifteen-story building that houses the Faculty of Medicine, Health Sciences Library, classrooms, laboratories, lecture halls, and a cafeteria.

Objectives: The Can$825,000 renovation project focused on several objectives including resolving environment, security, and access including lack of security from fire and theft; lack of climate control; lack of space; and restricted hours of access to the circulating collection.

Methods: The library was emptied before construction started. Rare materials were stored in secure off-site storage. Circu-

This was truly a cooperative project and could not have been accomplished without the hard work of many McGill staff, architects, consultants, contractors, and artisans. Staff from the Health Sciences Library, Library Technical Services, and the Department of Rare Books and Special Collections provided endless cheerful assistance. David Crawford, whose initial planning ensured a smooth-running project, kindly read this chapter and made many constructive suggestions. Stefan Michalski generously verified the technical information on conservation issues found here.

lating books were boxed and stored in the McIntyre Medical Sciences Building. During construction every part of the library except the two heritage rooms was gutted.

Results: Following three years of planning and eight months of renovations, the circulating collection opened as planned in September 2002. Rare books, reference, and archives opened in December 2002, one month later than planned. The results include security from fire and theft, manageable climate control, additional workspace, room to expand for years to come, and greater access to current collections.

Conclusions: This highly successful retrofit distinguished itself by the harmonious cooperation among several levels of expertise, from the Board of Curators to the project workers. The project is an example within the university's library system.

INTRODUCTION

In late November 2002, the Osler Library of the History of Medicine reopened its facilities with almost totally reconfigured spaces, heritage and nonheritage in design. Support from the Board of Curators and a generous private donation provided the impetus for a complicated retrofit which stressed a low-tech approach to the architecture and tight cooperation among the many departments and workers involved. The results include security from fire and theft, manageable climate control, additional workspace, room to expand for years to come, and greater access to current collections. The project is an example within the university library system.

Setting

The library comprises a collection of over 50,000 volumes whose basis is the original 8,000 donated by Sir William Osler. The Osler Library has an additional 14,000 rare books, spanning a time period from before the invention of printing to 1914, transferred from the McGill Health Sciences Library, which were donated or purchased since 1929. The library also has over 1,359 linear feet of archives including photographs, prints, and drawings, and has about 600 artifacts. In addition to these rare or fragile items, which are kept in locked stacks accessible only to library staff, the library has over 33,000 more recent volumes that can be borrowed and consulted by visitors. About 800 current and 50 rare items are added each year (see Photo 2.1).

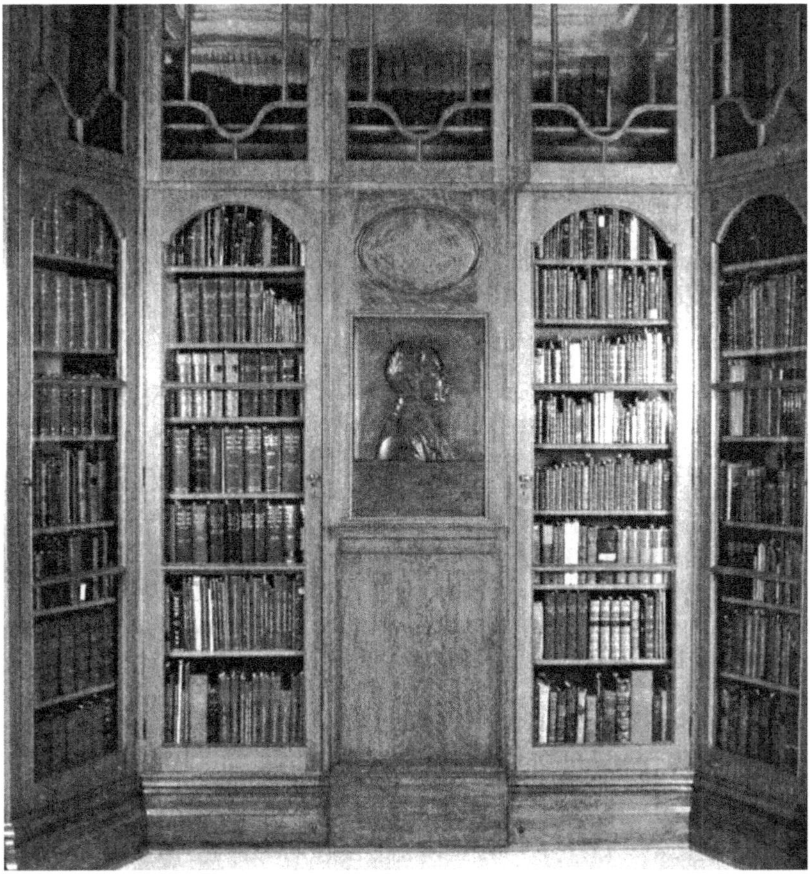

PHOTO 2.1. Profile of Sir William Osler by F. Vernon in the Osler Room. Photograph by Karen Coshof, 1979. Reprinted with permission.

History of the Library

Some information about the history of the library is necessary in order to understand this complicated retrofit. The Osler Library is important to McGill University both as an amazing scholarly resource and as an architectural masterpiece. It was opened with great ceremony in May 1929. The Chancellor of the University, Edward Beatty, presided. The Principal, Prime Minister of Canada, Dean of the McGill Medical Faculty, Vice-Rector of the University of Montreal, Professor W. S. Thayer of Johns Hopkins University, and the Very Reverend Arthur Carlisle, Anglican Dean and Rector of Montreal, completed the platform party. Harvey Cushing, renowned neurosurgeon and Osler's biographer, was among the distinguished guests and family members.[1] The library is unique among the libraries at McGill University, as it is partially governed by a Board of Curators, whose support proved essential in this undertaking.

The Osler Library was originally constructed inside the Strathcona Medical Building, which housed the Faculty of Medicine and the Medical—now Health Sciences—Library, the oldest medical library in Canada. The Strathcona Medical Building opened in 1911, replacing an earlier building that had been destroyed by fire in 1907. Most of the building and its contents, including the Medical Museum, were lost, but miraculously, not the library, which was protected by metal floors. The Osler Library was inserted into the Strathcona Medical Building, and Percy Erskine Nobbs, the son-in-law of William Osler's colleague and great friend, Professor of Anatomy, Francis J. Shepherd, designed the library to hold the almost 8,000 volumes of Osler's original donation. A 1930 description of the library written by Nobbs is featured in Appendix A.

The first Osler Librarian, Dr. W. W. Francis, Osler's cousin, was reluctant to add to the library's holdings. Annual board meetings became an agony for him as he attempted to maintain the library as a shrine to his beloved cousin, and resisted the urging of the board to spend money on books and journals.[2] The collection did, however, grow slowly and by 1963 numbered 17,500 volumes.

Dr. Francis died in 1959, around the same time as the Faculty of Medicine began planning a new medical building. The Osler Library clearly belonged adjacent to the Health Sciences Library and at the heart of the faculty, and the decision was made, late in the planning process, to move the entire Osler Library to a panhandle-shaped wing added to the still unfinished circular McIntyre Medical Sciences Building. This wing consists of two floors (third and fourth) and results in the Osler Library being "suspended" in the air and being exposed to the environment on all but one side. Funding for the move of the entire physical Osler Library was provided by the John and Mary R. Markle Foundation of New York. A new room, the Wellcome Camera, was designed by Neil J. Elliott, and added in recognition of the Wellcome Trust's generous support of the Osler's book purchases in the sterling area.[3]

The expansion and move of the library occurred as the faculty itself was expanding and just as the History of Medicine department was created. In 1966, when the new building and relocated Osler Library opened, Dr. Donald Bates was appointed as Professor of the History of Medicine and Acting Osler Librarian. This was an important appointment as Bates' vision included a dynamic research collection linked to a department made up of anthropologists, sociologists, and historians working on the interactions between medicine and society.[4] His vision guaranteed two important elements in the Osler Library: an increased budget for book purchases and a growing body of researchers and students. The Osler Library is unusual for a history of medicine library as its collection consists of both rare books and a large circulating collection of more modern secondary works.

Over the next thirty years, the History of Medicine department and the library, which shared the space, grew together. By the late 1990s it was clear that both the library and the department had outgrown their quarters. Due to the architectural importance of the library it was clear that it could not be moved again and its physical situation made expansion virtually impossible. The Department was relocated and the space was allocated to the library. The library occupied the 3,680 square-foot third floor and housed the Wellcome Camera (reference collection and research space for rare books, circulating material, and general study area), two rest rooms, and seating for eight researchers. Adjacent was the Osler Room, holding some of the circulating collection and exhibits and seating six researchers for general study. The Osler Room and the Wellcome Camera are both considered heritage rooms (see Figures 2.1 and 2.2).

The 3,594 square-foot fourth floor held 22,000 rare books including folio volumes on inappropriate shelving, packed tightly in three

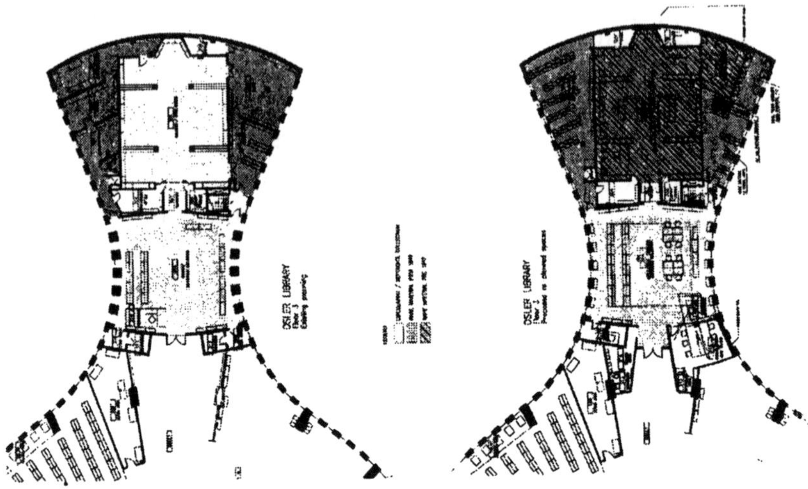

FIGURE 2.1. Osler Library third-floor renovation drawing. Reprinted with permission by Fournier Gersovitz Moss et associés architectes.

separate closed stack areas, the remainder of the circulating collection, and the archives (see Photo 2.2).

The Department of Social Studies of Medicine occupied about 2,260 square feet of the fourth floor. Their space consisted of faculty and graduate student offices, a kitchen, and a seminar room. Sharing space with staff and students made security a constant concern. Although the building had smoke detectors, it did not have a sprinkler system. Solid locks provided the only security to storage areas. Rare books and archives consultation took place in the Wellcome Camera, the general reference and reading area, making adequate supervision impossible. There were no lockers for bags. The library was closed evenings and weekends. Furthermore, the lack of climate control facilities suitable for rare books was becoming dangerous.

Once the Faculty of Medicine decided to relocate the department it was necessary to ensure the space released was allocated to the library, determine how the additional space should be used, and present outline plans to the Board of Curators. In November 1998, the board agreed to the broad outline and agreed that renovations to the library were a major funding priority. Based on very basic estimates, the cost was estimated at about Can$700,000.

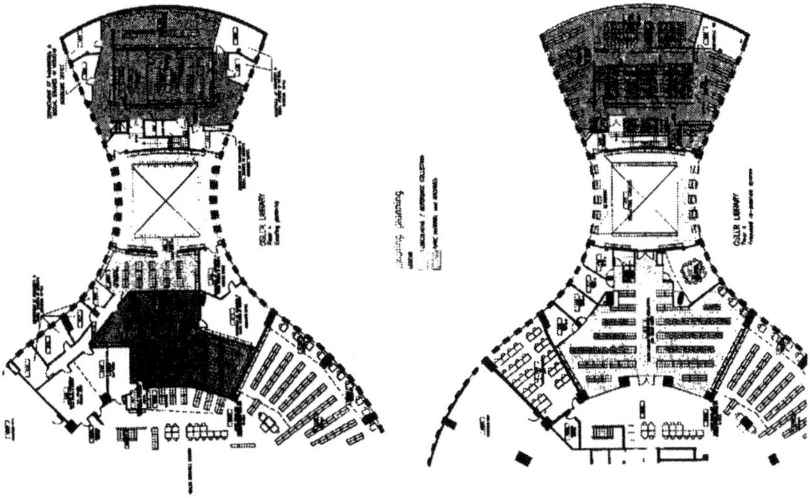

FIGURE 2.2. Osler Library fourth-floor renovation drawing. Reprinted with permission by Fournier Gersovitz Moss et associés architectes.

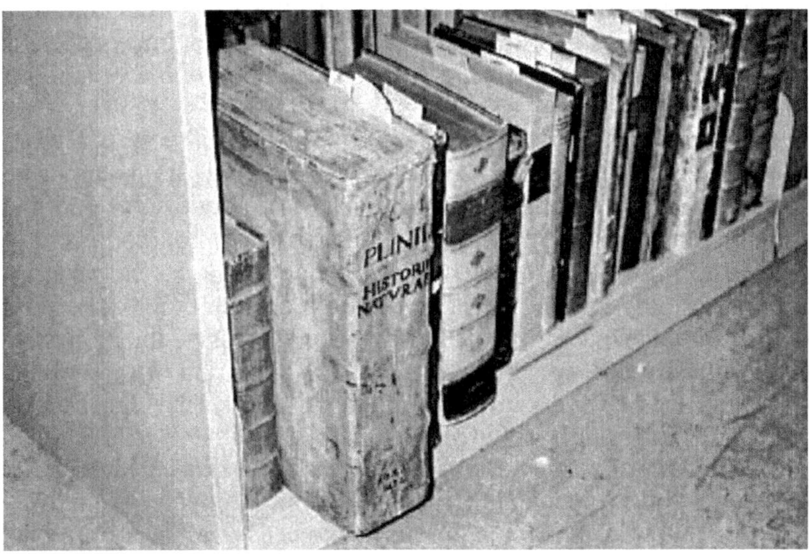

PHOTO 2.2. Prerenovation folio shelving. Reprinted with permission by Pamela Miller.

One of the Osler Library's most avid supporters is the Dean of Medicine and Chair of the Board of Curators, Dr. Abraham Fuks. Fuks approached Dr. John McGovern, a noted allergist from Texas and one of the founders of the American Osler Society. McGovern generously donated US$350,000. The university allocated 2,055 square feet of the departmental space to the library. McGill University librarian David Crawford then worked to ensure the Osler Library renovation was placed on the university's list of renovation priorities. Fuks convinced the university to contribute approximately Can$300,000 toward the project. In addition, Crawford and Fuks were able to get the university to reroof and rehabilitate the external "shell" of the panhandle so that "the project" was restricted to internal renovations.

Objectives

The building project focused on several objectives including environment, security, and access. Climate control suitable for rare books had to be introduced into a 1960s building that was poorly designed to handle the Montreal climate—which swings from more than thirty degrees centigrade in the summer to minus thirty degrees centigrade in the winter. Fire and theft protection needed to be improved. The journal and circulating book collections needed to be available for longer hours.

Crawford drew up the initial broad outlines of how the space should be reconfigured, recommending that all the rare materials be concentrated at the far end of the panhandle on both floors and that the library offices, journals, and circulating collection be moved to the fourth floor. This arrangement would allow for special environmental controls for the rare material and place the Osler circulating collection adjacent to the Health Sciences Library—thus allowing evening and weekend access. Crawford's suggestion of moving the library offices solved another problem as their former location no longer met the requirements of the fire code.

The board was particularly keen to hire an experienced heritage architect for this project and their support helped convince the university that this was as much a "heritage project" as a renovation one. The university thus engaged Julia Gersovitz, of Fournier, Gersovitz and Moss Associates for the project. Gersovitz is an architect who is well-known for her work on heritage buildings in Montreal and elsewhere. At her invitation, Stefan Michalski, Head of Preventive Conservation Services at the Canadian Conservation Institute (CCI), acted as consultant. Michalski inspected the rare books and advised that the main conservation problems were the threat of fire, lack of adequate security, and the inability to control fluctuations in temperature and humidity. After meeting with library staff, investigating the original plans of the library, and verifying building dimensions and shelving requirements, the architects drew up a report.[5] In November 2000, Gersovitz presented her preliminary report to the curators who combed over it and made useful suggestions, which were incorporated into the plans. One example was that the environmental control unit should be accessible to maintenance technicians at all times and therefore not located in a secure area, and not situated above a collection.

Relative Humidity

The most important change to the library's original plan for the rare book collection came during a roundtable discussion with all parties present: the conservation scientist adviser (Michalski), the architect (Gersovitz), and the librarians. During this discussion, it became evident that a "simple" solution of providing 50 percent relative humidity (RH) everywhere was not feasible for various reasons, including the budgetary implications of modifying exterior walls and the threat to the historic integrity of the Osler Room. Michalski noted that books have different humidity requirements. Although a book with rag paper and a parchment or skin binding is best served by a 50 percent RH, an acidic paper book with case binding is best served by a lower RH. The only common ground was that dampness (over 75 percent RH) was to be avoided for all books, at all costs. He noted that a practical boundary could be drawn between the two groups of humidity requirements at the year of manufacture of 1840, this being the approximate date at which alum-rosin sizing and wood pulp began to dominate paper production, and thus the date beyond which books were more likely to be acidic.

A practical solution emerged from these discussions, which merged knowledge of the components of the collections, available spaces, and competing humidity issues. The Osler Room could accommodate the 12,000 volumes published before 1840, and with no exterior walls, it could be maintained at a constant 50 percent RH and be serviced by its own climate control unit. The remaining spaces in the panhandle with their exterior walls would hold the post-1840 books. The heating and ventilating for this post-1840 area could be adapted to the existing building system. The systems would be improved for stability, but the RH in winter would not be maintained at a value that threatened the walls. The result would be that the post-1840 material would benefit from the slightly drier, cooler winter atmosphere. Michalski did not consider this RH fluctuation between winter and summer to be a significant risk to this group of books. Elimination of the extreme summer fluctuations, particularly high RH that had been caused by mechanical system inadequacies of the past, was important. By adapting to the design of the building and eliminating the need for a vapor barrier on the exterior walls, the architect decreased the project costs dramatically. And by keeping the mechanical systems relatively uncomplicated and reliable, the risk of system malfunction that Michalski had seen result in mold in collections, would be much reduced.

Gersovitz summarized the project as a low-tech approach that capitalized on the unusual history of the Osler Library, and the image of the Osler Room as a cocoon. The project was described as respectful of the Osler Room's heritage, and as a means to reestablish its fundamental importance to the Osler Library. The approach and conservation design guidelines used were sanctioned by the CCI. As the plans met the budget, the project was realizable, in part because of the use of the Osler Room, and in the downscaling of the RH targets.[6]

METHODS

For reasons of clarity, important planning steps used in this renovation project are listed in Appendix B and highlights are discussed briefly here. Consultation and cooperation are important concepts in the success of this renovation project. Since moving a library requires collection knowledge, it was helpful that David Crawford had worked with library staff for several years to ensure that the whole of the Osler Library's print collections were fully cataloged and available online. Subsequently, location changes to the online catalog proceeded fairly smoothly. It was fortunate that McGill University's Department of Facilities Development assigned a renovation project manager who had a consultative style. On-site weekly meetings took place throughout the renovation process, attended by the history of medicine librarian, project manager, architect, foreman, and specialists such as electricians, ventilation engineers, and fire detection experts. Minutes were taken and circulated, essential for remembering decisions made about particular questions. Meetings were always pleasant, and sometimes hilarious. Retrofits can be full of surprises and this project was no exception. During one meeting the only way of knowing if an existing passageway could be widened was for the foreman to take his sledgehammer and demolish the masonry on the spot. Similarly, despite detailed plans, it was important to be present at meetings to make final decisions such as the locations of computer outlets or light switches.

The history of medicine librarian was previously involved in a major expansion of a museum. This project proved to be a beneficial experience, the most important lesson of which was that the impossible *could* be done. One of the most helpful books at the time was Elizabeth Habich's *Moving Library Collections: A Management Handbook.* She states that no one over age forty should be involved in physically packing and moving the books.[7] That advice eliminated all three Osler Library staff, who then were made responsible only for physically packing the contents of their own offices. Habich also stressed the importance of public relations.

Osler Library decided to hire a "move manager" and was fortunate to "borrow" a McGill Law Library staff member who had managed their recent move. The move manager was given a twelve-month contract to manage all the details connected with packing, shipping, unpacking, and reshelving. The move manager and his staff calculated the amount of time needed to pack the collection (see Appendix C).

In all, nineteen students and contract employees were hired as packers, including two museology technicians. The role of the museology technicians was to train and supervise those packing the rare books to take special care with fragile items. An additional reason for engaging specialists is that a move can be a golden opportunity to do a little preventive conservation, as some of the protection prepared for the fragile books can be designed to remain with the books permanently (see Photo 2.3).

During lulls in the packing process, time was spent preparing simple acid-free paper book jackets for journals that had disintegrating

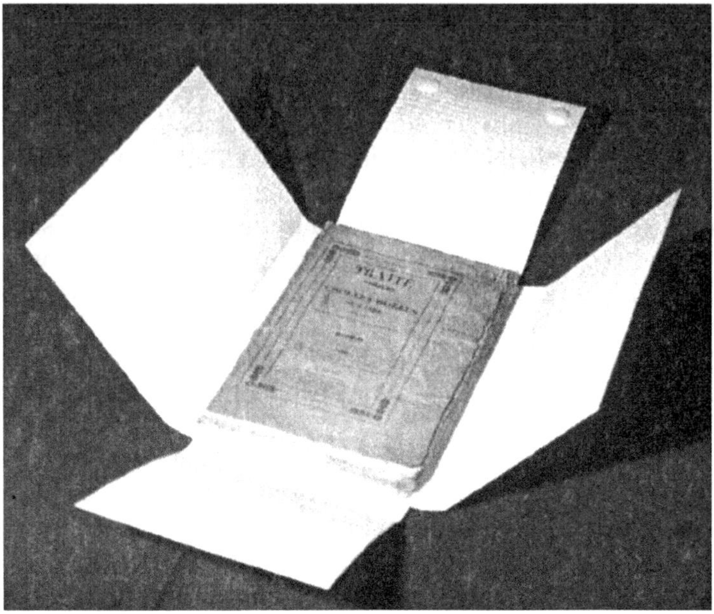

PHOTO 2.3. Conservation packing designed to remain with the book. Reprinted with permission by Pamela Miller.

leather bindings. This is an inexpensive, safe, and relatively durable solution to stabilizing the covers of books that are unlikely to be restored.

Moving and Storage

The library had to be empty before construction could begin. Secure off-site storage for rare material was rented. To avoid rapid changes in temperature or humidity, the rare material could not be transported during extremes of weather. The circulating books were also boxed and were stored elsewhere in the McIntyre Medical Sciences Building. The entire project had to be carried out without unnecessarily disrupting the academic requirements of professorial staff and students. Due to noise concerns, construction ceased during examination times. Quebec has a mandatory two-week construction holiday in July. To reduce the number of volumes to be packed, McGill Library staff, who are entitled to borrow sixty books, were strongly encouraged to do so. Graduate student borrowing limits were raised to sixty books for the duration of the renovation period. The Department of Rare Books and Special Collections at McGill University's central library agreed to house the rare material that researchers had requested to be put aside for their work during the summer months, for once material was packed it could not be retrieved. After much publicity, the library closed in mid-March and started the packing process. Book packers worked in shifts from 9:00 a.m. to 5:00 p.m. The entire collection was packed, shipped, and/or stored well before construction began in early May.

During construction every part of the library except the two heritage rooms was gutted. Because the library wanted to ensure that circulating materials were available for students at the beginning of September, work was completed in this area first. All areas of the library were fitted with a sophisticated smoke detection and sprinkler system. Electrical wiring was upgraded. Low ultraviolet (UV) lighting was installed in the reading and storage areas. Windows in the storage areas were covered by blackout blinds affixed to the frames with Velcro. Great pains were taken to remove or upgrade defective or unnecessary pipes, drains, and vents, which had been sources of random leaks.

The smoke detectors and sprinklers in the heritage rooms were designed to be as unobtrusive as possible. After the plasterwork was repaired, these rooms were repainted. The original glass doors on the Osler Room cabinets had been removed and stored in 1966 when the room had been designated for the circulating collection. These glass doors were repaired and placed back on the shelving units.

Project Compromises

Due to the security system and the requirements of the environmental control unit, the Osler Room (pre-1840 books) has unavoidably become a locked vault. This means that library visitors may no longer study in it, nor view the display case now housed there unless they are accompanied by a staff member. Recollections of studying in this inspirational area are dear to many visitors. The room, however, is effectively lighted, with low level, UV-filtered lights and is always visible through glass entrance doors. Although installing glass doors on rare book bookcases is not generally recommended due to the potential creation of microclimates, in this situation, vents are located in each door and alarm contacts on these doors serve as extra security during visits to the Osler Room. This room is still a destination point for Oslerians and visitors. Four new exhibition cases were designed by Robert Anderson to give the rare books more visibility.

RESULTS

The circulating collection opened as planned on September 3, 2002. Rare book, reference, and archives opened on December 2, 2002, one month later than planned. The delay was caused by the need to link the Osler Library's security system with university security, and to change OPAC location fields to reflect the separation of rare books published before and after 1840.

The renovation project's results surpassed the library's expectations. Seating for regular study was increased from fourteen to sixteen. Previously, there was no seating dedicated to rare book research. Ten places are divided between two rooms, one for consulting pre-1840 and the other for post-1840 books. Overall shelving space was increased, especially with the use of compact shelving.

The two climate-controlled storage areas were thoroughly tested during dramatic swings in temperature in recent seasons. The improved conditions were seen almost immediately in the pre-1840 collection, with vellum-covered books losing their brittle look and feel. The new controls make it possible to maintain the RH at 40 percent and the heat at twenty degrees centigrade in the Osler Room (pre-1840). Extremely efficient air filters throughout the rare book and archive storage have eliminated almost all dust. Particles of greasy black soot no longer seep through the vents. The W. W. Francis Seminar Room has been relocated and is slightly smaller, seating sixteen persons. Staff appreciate their own new offices and new furniture, which are designed to accommodate computers. Overall, the collections are much easier to work with, as there is space for expansion and room for staff to move around easily while retrieving material. A huge advantage is that the journal and circulating book collections are now accessible on evenings and weekends.

New security measures include motion detectors, card-reader access to storage areas, and supervised glass-fronted rare book and archive research rooms with camera surveillance. Researchers are asked to leave their bags in lockers that have library-provided locks.

The well-attended reopening ceremony featured speakers who paid tribute to McGovern's generosity and recognized his vision by unveiling a stained glass window that incorporated his portrait. This window shares space with other windows bearing the arms of Canadian universities that have medical faculties. Finally, the Osler Library is proud to say that this project has set new standards in conservation for McGill University's other outstanding rare book collections.

APPENDIX A: THE WORDS OF THE ARCHITECT

In the words of Percy Nobbs, the architect of the Osler Library:

> These ancient volumes are of course of extraordinary human, scientific and literary interest, but a large percentage of them are also works of art, being exquisitely printed and sumptuously bound. The shelves thus present a charming colour scheme of vellum, calf and dyed leathers, and in the design of the Osler Library at McGill everything has been subordinated to the books themselves which are arranged in full view, behind glazed doors.
>
> Four structural columns occur in the room, which is lined in oak, or glazed bookcasing throughout, up to the level of their capitals. The columns divide the Library into three bays on either side, with a central aisle having the entrance doors at the one end and at the other a niche. In this there is a fine bronze portrait panel of the late Sir William Osler by F. Vernon, under which there is a secret receptacle for the casket [containing the ashes of Sir William Osler] above alluded to. The original design of the room, with a barrel vault across the centre bays, in which there is a skylight, has not been interfered with. Besides this top light, there are three windows in leaded glazing with devices in grisaille work. Flanking the centre window and in the lunette opposite are the arms of the six institutions of learning with which the great physician was most intimately connected—Toronto, McGill, Pennsylvania, Johns Hopkins, Oxford and Christchurch—together with his own heraldic achievement. . . . The fitting up of the room is the work of The Bromsgrove Guild of Canada, and very great pains were taken to secure a finish which, without any suspicion of artificial patination, succeeds in bringing out the full damask effect of the chamf of the quartered oak in velvet brown tones.
>
> The floor is covered with haircloth, over felt, and on this are strewn a notably harmonious collection of Kazak rugs of sunburst pattern in mulberry reds and ivory white.

The furniture is in oak to match the wainscot work and while frankly inspired by old English models, is of no particular period. Here, as elsewhere, the intention has been to do things simply and solidly, in the hope that all may go on growing old together gracefully, as the saying is, with the books on the shelves.

The fittings and furnishings of the Osler Library were designed by Messrs. Nobbs & Hyde, Architects, of Montreal.[8]

APPENDIX B: STEPS IN THE PLANNING PROCESS

1. Prepare an outline draft plan.
2. Consult publications and experts.
3. Discuss the plan with all interested parties—the Board of Curators, the Department of Social Studies of Medicine, the Department of Facilities Development, and the University Planning Office in particular.
4. Revise the plan to meet most of the perceived needs.
5. Hire an experienced architect and project manager to draw up detailed plans.
6. Work closely with the experts to hire experienced and reliable contractors.

Public Relations

- Establish a flowchart to keep everyone on track and reassure staff and library users.
- Limit inconvenience to academic staff and students by issuing advanced information of the project; increasing borrowing limits; housing needed rare research material in a suitable library; and advising professors of the wisdom of scheduling courses to accommodate unforeseen delays. Inform general public through the use of Web pages, notes on mailing lists, messages on the OPAC, information in *Osler Library Newsletter*, and footers on e-mails. A virtual exhibition of the project was added to the Osler Library Web page, which included new pictures as the project evolved.
- Establish clear deadlines, in writing, and note constraints such as requesting that all construction noise cease during examinations.
- Inform the building manager and the adjacent Health Sciences Library about construction requirements (and interruptions) in terms of use of loading dock and freight elevator.

Storage

Locate climate-controlled secure storage suitable for rare books and archives. The circulating collection and library furniture (excluding metal shelving) were stored in the McIntyre Building and in the adjacent Health Sciences Library as that library was not as busy during the summer months. One thirteen-foot, oak bookshelf from Norham Gardens (Osler's residence in Oxford), was shrink-wrapped for additional protection. Metal shelving units were stored off-site, but on campus.

Packing Processes

- Hire additional, experienced staff, for supervisory roles, technical expertise, packing, unpacking, and reshelving.
- Purchase supplies and be sure to give suppliers time to fill the order or use several suppliers to avoid running out of material. Some companies sell "seconds" (slightly damaged boxes or with faulty lettering) at reduced prices.
- Prepare collections for packing. Although great efforts had been made in the last decade to fully catalog the printed collections, this was an excellent opportunity to tidy up loose ends. The contract of a temporary archivist was extended to ensure that all items in the collection were boxed and correctly labeled.
- Relocate library staff to suitable accommodations and identify regular work and/or projects that can be carried out during relocation.

Transport

- Engage a specialized transport company after checking references and comparing bids.
- Inform the University Security Department that a chase car will be needed to follow each rare book shipment to the storage destination, and once the project was completed, to follow each shipment back.

Location Changes

- Arrange with Library Technical Services to have personnel on the spot to make online catalog location changes as books were unpacked prior to reshelving. This process also acted as a valuable way to inventory the rare collection.

APPENDIX C: GUIDELINES USED TO CALCULATE PACKING AND UNPACKING TIME

Packing

Note: Each rare book was wrapped in tissue.

- Circulating books: 20 books per box (10" × 15½" × 12½")
- Rare books: 12 books per box (10" × 15½" × 12 ½")

Time

- One hundred eighty-three boxes of circulating books were packed per day by a workforce of eight packers working constantly in shifts.
- Twenty-four boxes of rare books were packed per day by a workforce of two museum technicians and two to three students working constantly in shifts.

Unpacking

- Four persons worked full-time for ten days to unpack the circulating books.
- Three to four experienced staff worked full-time to input location changes for the rare books.
- Three to four persons unpacked and divided the collection at 1840, took the books to catalogers, and reshelved the books after the location changes were made in the catalog.

NOTES

1. Davey, Lycurgus. "Harvey Cushing and the Humanities in Medicine." *Journal of the History of Medicine and Allied Sciences* 24(April 1969): 119-124.

2. Bliss, Michael. *William Osler: A Life in Medicine*. Toronto: University of Toronto Press, 1999: 492.

3. Stevenson, Lloyd G. "The Translation of the Osler Library from the Strathcona Building to the McIntyre Building." *Osler Library Newsletter* 14(October 1973): 2.

4. Wallis, Faith and Miller, Pamela. "A Tribute: Dr. Don G. Bates." *Osler Library Newsletter* 96(2001): 6-7.

5. Fournier, Gersovitz Moss et associés architectes. *The Osler Library of the History of Medicine McGill University, Report on the Proposed Renovation*, 2000.

6. Michalski, Stefan. *Guidelines for Humidity and Temperature for Canadian Archives.* Ottawa, Ontario: Canadian Conservation Institute Technical Bulletin 23, 2000.

7. Habich, Elizabeth. *Moving Library Collections: A Management Handbook.* Westport, CT: Greenwood Press, 1998: 118.

8. Nobbs, Percy E. "Bibliotheca Osleriana—McGill University, Montreal." *The Journal, Royal Architectural Institute of Canada* 6(June 1930): 204.

PART II: HOSPITAL LIBRARIES

Case Study 3

Booker Health Sciences Library

Catherine M. Boss

OVERVIEW

Setting: Jersey Shore University Medical Center, a 502-bed teaching hospital, had a remotely located medical library and a school of nursing library housed in the basement of a former office building behind the Medical Center.

Objectives: Project objectives included planning and building a new library in a highly visible area; and consolidating the medical and nursing library collections, and a new consumer health collection.

Methods: The Coordinator of Library Services developed a concept plan for a new library that outlined collection, shelving, seating, technology, and staff requirements and projected a space need of 5,000 square feet. Cost estimate for the project was $1.3 million, which included relocation costs for the existing departments in the planned space. Funding for the project needed to be found from outside sources.

Results: The Booker Health Sciences Library was constructed at a cost of $1.5 million, funded in its entirety with private monies. The library is window-lined, furnished with cherrywood, and easily accessible for staff and the public. A single customer service area serves as the focal point for both staff and the public. Features include areas for quiet study, leisure reading, and collaborative work.

Conclusions: The new Booker Health Sciences Library brought together three distinct components of health care information—medicine, nursing, and consumer health—into a library that has beauty and functionality.

INTRODUCTION

Jersey Shore University Medical Center, formerly Jersey Shore Medical Center, is located in Monmouth County, New Jersey, two miles from the ocean. The Medical Center is a 502-bed full service facility with a complement of 700 physicians and 3,500 employees. It offers fully approved residency programs in general dentistry, internal medicine, pediatrics, preliminary medicine, obstetrics and gynecology, and general surgery; and fellowships in primary care sports medicine, geriatrics, and infectious diseases. A multiplicity of students in medicine, nursing, pharmacy, social work, psychology, physician assistant, premedicine, and pastoral care programs participate in clinical rotations and internships. The Medical Center was renamed Jersey Shore University Medical Center in June 2003, to better reflect its status as an academic medical center and university affiliate.

Library Services

The Booker Health Sciences Library project was completed prior to the name change, so this case study will use the former name. Prior to 1997, library services were segregated. A medical library in the hospital proper provided library services for physicians and house staff. The school of nursing's library provided services for nursing students, faculty, and nurses. The location and ambience of these libraries shared similarities, but their service missions varied greatly.

The medical library was located on the second floor of the Medical Center in a remote area adjacent to the on-call rooms for obstetrics/gynecology residents. The library was not easily accessible. There were no directional signs directing people to it, nor was the library included on the directional maps for visitors. New employees were not told of its location during orientation. The primary mission of the medical library was to serve the needs of physicians and house staff. Nurses and employees were led to believe this library and its resources were not available to them.

The medical library facility covered 2,541 square feet, with two large rooms separated by a sliding glass door. One side housed the circulating book collection, reference book collection, reference desk, director's office, and four study carrels, two of which had a computer workstation. The other room housed the current journal collection, bound journal collection in an alcove that was not wheelchair accessible, small book collection of core medical texts for night use, and twelve study carrels, two of which had a computer workstation. The sliding glass door between the two rooms was locked at the end of the business day. Physicians, house staff, and nursing supervisors could gain access to this journal room after hours using a security badge access system.

The medical library had painted cinder block walls, mismatched furniture, and linoleum flooring. A circulation/reference desk was there, but workspace for library staff was inadequate. The ambience and functionality of the medical library needed to be renovated and upgraded if the library was to grow and change its service role.

The Ann May School of Nursing was a diploma nursing school operated by Jersey Shore Medical Center from 1905 through 1998 and located in an office complex behind the Medical Center. The 3,306 square-foot library was located in the basement of the building, accessible only by a long, steep stairway. The library had no elevator access, which made it inaccessible to the physically disabled. The basement location provided its own set of environmental issues. Because the building was built on a dried-up lake, water leaked into the library during periods of heavy rain. Termites swarmed each spring and the library frequently smelled of sewage. The mechanical room for the building was located next to the library, creating a noise distraction. In spite of its location and persistent environmental issues, the library had a strong service mission. The library, although primarily serving the curricular needs of the school of nursing, was open to everyone.

Possible Merger of Libraries

The idea of merging these two library facilities had been discussed for more than twenty years. In the fall of 1984, Medical Center administration, with a deep sense of commitment to achieving excellence as a major teaching hospital, commissioned a consultant to identify and help develop the resources necessary to provide the essential educational support services at a level to commensurate with teaching facilities. An administrative merger of the two libraries was recommended. A preliminary space planning study was done by the Medical Center's architectural firm. Directors of both libraries felt the presented plans were inadequate and did not reflect their collections or services. Hospital and nursing school archives storage, computer facilities for patrons, microfilm service, audiovisual services, consumer health services, and projected library expansions were not included. Plans to merge the two libraries were shelved.

Over the next ten years, personnel changes in both libraries and workplace design throughout the Medical Center resulted in the elimination of the medical library director position. Staffing for the medical library was outsourced and talks of merging the two libraries rekindled.

A 1995 report by the Pew Health Professions Commission recommended that the "size and number of nursing education programs be reduced, due to a loss of perhaps 60 percent of hospital beds."[1] This report was a precursor to a pivotal decision made by the Medical Center's Board of Trustees to close the Ann May School of Nursing in June 1998. Fewer job opportunities, coupled with the uncertainty of federal reimbursement, prompted the decision. This decision heightened efforts to build a new health sciences library that would merge the two libraries, but was slowed down slightly by the decision to merge Jersey Shore Medical Center with the Medical Center of Ocean County and Riverview Medical Center to form the Meridian Health System.

HEALTH SCIENCES LIBRARY PLANNING

In 1997, the Vice President for Academic Affairs, James McCorkel, PhD, embarked on a mission to endow and construct a comprehensive, up-to-date health sciences library. In presenting his mission to administration, he declared that a new library was imperative to prepare for the health care challenges of the future, concurring with the 1984 consultant report. The library would symbolize the Medical Center's commitment to the professional development and growth of its nursing and medical staff. A consumer health resource center within the library would make quality books, periodicals, and databases available to patients and the community.

Key to the success of the project was the hiring of a Senior Library Coordinator in May 1997. Catherine M. Boss, library coordinator, had twenty-four years experience in the profession, including the orchestration of a similar nursing/medical library merger. The coordinator immediately prepared for the Booker project by familiarizing herself with the Medical Center's operating and capital budget processes, reading about current library construction projects, and visiting new libraries in the state.

The project's first challenge was finding a location that met projected space needs. In extrapolating these space needs, four assumptions were made:

1. The level of customer use would increase. Library use by staff nurses would increase because of its new on-site location. The number of medical students rotating to Jersey Shore would also increase as the Medical Center's affiliation with the Robert Wood Johnson Medical School strengthened. Increased research within the Medical Center would precipitate increased library use. A new consumer health collection would attract patients, patient families, and the public to the library.
2. Information seekers would increasingly demand library resources in electronic format at their desktops. Space for library collections would have to be as flexible as possible to ensure maximum functionality. Greater emphasis should be on access to the collections rather than storage.
3. Librarians would spend increasingly greater time educating customers on informatics and on how to find quality information on the Internet. Space for mediated teaching and learning workstations would be needed.
4. Customers would visit the library for quiet contemplation and professional comportment.

With these assumptions in mind, a concept plan for the new library was developed. The plan outlined collection, shelving, seating, technology, and staff requirements, following established guidelines and a formula for library space planning.[2] A net-space requirement of 5,000 square feet was projected for the library's collections, customers, and staff. The plan recommended the use of high-density shelving to house the combined collections.

August 1997 marked a milestone in the project when Medical Center administration authorized $10,000 to be spent for Phase 1 design services by their architectural firm. Phase 1 called for the development of a space and facilities program for the new library, identification of potential locations within the Jersey Shore facility plan, and cost estimates for construction. The money, however, came with a caveat from administration. Given the growing need for financial resources for the evolving Meridian system, capital funds would not be committed to construction. The construction could proceed only with substantial outside support.

Phase 1 did not proceed without issue. Literature has shown that participation by the librarian in the planning process is essential for a well-planned, functional library that is responsive to space needs.[3] In addition to detailing the space requirements, a design plan should incorporate the library staff's philosophy of service.[4] This philosophy directly affects the functionality of the space planned and plays a major role in the success or failure of the finished library.

The library's involvement with the architectural firm ended with the concept plan for a new library. The firm did not consult with library staff about their service philosophy or dreams of what the new library should be like. The firm did consult via telephone with the director of the George F. Smith Library, University of Medicine and Dentistry of New Jersey, to gain some perspective on library planning.

In October 1997 the architectural firm presented two design plans, one for 4,200 square feet and the other for 3,500 square feet. A location on the first floor of the Booker Pavilion, adjacent to the visitor's parking lot, was recommended. The location would be accessible and its window-lined wall would make the library visible from the visitors' parking lot. Although both plans were acceptable in terms of location, they were unacceptable with respect to size and functionality. A recommendation was made to administration to obtain the services of a new architectural firm with experience in designing health sciences libraries. This recommendation came to fruition in an indirect way when a change in leadership at the Medical Center resulted in the hiring of a new architectural firm, Granary Associates.

Early in 1998, Granary began working on a master plan for the Medical Center that included space for a new health sciences library. Granary also recommended the Booker location and a library of just under 5,000 square feet, a size that was close to the concept design. Cost for the project was set at $1.3 million, entailing four phases:

Phase 1: Relocation of all offices occupying the Booker One South location and the northern offices of the Booker One North location.

Phase 2: Renovation of the vacated Booker One North area and relocation of the Human Resources Department to this renovated area.

Phase 3: Renovation of the vacated Human Resources area and relocation of the chapel from the Booker South location to Booker North.

Phase 4: Renovation of the vacant Booker South area for the library, redesign of the Booker lobby, and construction of a workroom for pastoral care volunteers.

Granary's proposal was approved, but could not begin until outside funding was found.

Meanwhile, May 1998 brought the closing of the school of nursing and a decision to merge the two libraries on a limited basis. The nursing library's services coordinator joined the merged library staff. A core collection of books, a ten-year backfile of the nursing journals and the nursing card catalog were set up in an alcove of the journal room in the medical library. Administration decided that the remaining collection could remain in the old nursing library until the new library was built, confident that private monies would be found to build the library. Through all types of weather, library staff and a security escort traveled back and forth to the old nursing library to obtain needed materials.

PROJECT FINANCING

Financing of the project was the next concern. To accomplish this, a partnership needed to be cultivated with the Foundation Office. A telephone call was made to Paulette Roberts, the foundation's director, during her first week on the job. The library project was promoted in great detail and depicted as a great opportunity for a first major fund-raising campaign. This created a sense of ownership by the foundation for the project. A formal presentation on the proposed library was made to the foundation's board of directors in September 1998.

Concurrently, Medical Center administration committed to begin the project when $800,000 had been raised. Granary spent time with the library staff to gain perspective on their vision for a new library, get a feel for the ambience and style of library that was envisioned (warm and inviting; more traditional than contemporary), and learn about customer service points that needed to be included:

- Segregated technology center with systems librarians office nearby
- Centrally located customer service desk
- Separate journal reading areas for physicians, nurses, and consumers
- Separate carrel and table study areas
- Segregated, enclosed photoduplication area
- Segregated telephone area to facilitate patient confidentiality
- Storage for nursing school and hospital archives
- Microfilm intershelved with bound volumes
- Consumer health area
- Segregated work area for staff

Discussions with the architects and foundation personnel were successful. The Foundation Office, in partnership with the library, was able to raise all monies needed for the project through private sources, with the naming opportunity coming from the Jane H. and J. Marshall Booker Charitable Foundation. Major contributors to the project included The Mildred H. Rosa Charitable Trust Foundation; Jean and Don Lass; $100,000 in contributions from Jersey Shore's medical/dental staff; and the nursing staff and alumni of the Ann May School of Nursing, who contributed over $32,000 in a six-week "Nurses for Knowledge" pledge campaign.

With funding secured, work began in mid-1999 to finalize the library's floor plan and interior design features. Granary, the hospital's Manager of Plant Operations, and library staff met regularly to decide on wood finishes, wall colors, carpeting, and the like. Granary preselected several colors and patterns for staff selection. To create the desired ambience, cherrywood was selected for the crown and baseboard molding; colonial blue, plum, and off-white colors for the walls; and patterned carpeting with solid accent carpeting for the customer service, carrel, and table areas. Meetings were also held with the telecommunications and information technology departments to design the computer infrastructure and telecommunications system for the facility. New computers were requested through the capital budget process (see Figure 3.1).

FURNISHINGS

Interior furnishings were the next concern. High-density electronic shelving was identified to house the combined collections, and chosen as it provided the highest safety measures for 24/7 after-hours access. This shelving's end paneling would match the cherrywood crown and baseboard molding of the cantilever book and journal display shelving. Cherry study carrels, and tables with black fireslate countertops were selected to complete the interior.

Since sturdy cherry library chairs were not found, oak chairs were ordered unfinished and stained cherry to match the carrels and tables. To select the lounge seating, the library coordinator made a field trip to Granary headquarters in Philadelphia and test-sat several models. Because the design of the customer service area did not lend itself to manufactured furniture, the service desk was custom-made of cherrywood with a green Corian countertop.

After an extensive process, bids were awarded in June 2000. Substantial savings were realized by contracting with Arnold Geisler to custom-build the study tables, carrels, end paneling, and crown and baseboard molding. By slightly redesigning the carrel, Geisler was able to add two additional carrels in each section. Prior to the awarding of bids, a trip was made to Geisler's manufacturing plant to see how the furniture would be made.

PREPARATION OF THE NURSING COLLECTION

To prepare the nursing collection for integration, duplication and outdated materials were weeded out. The nursing collection was reclassified from the Dewey decimal classification scheme to the National Library of Medicine system. From February through April 2000, each library staff member worked from home one day a week with a batch of shelf list cards, reclassifying, and ordering bar codes

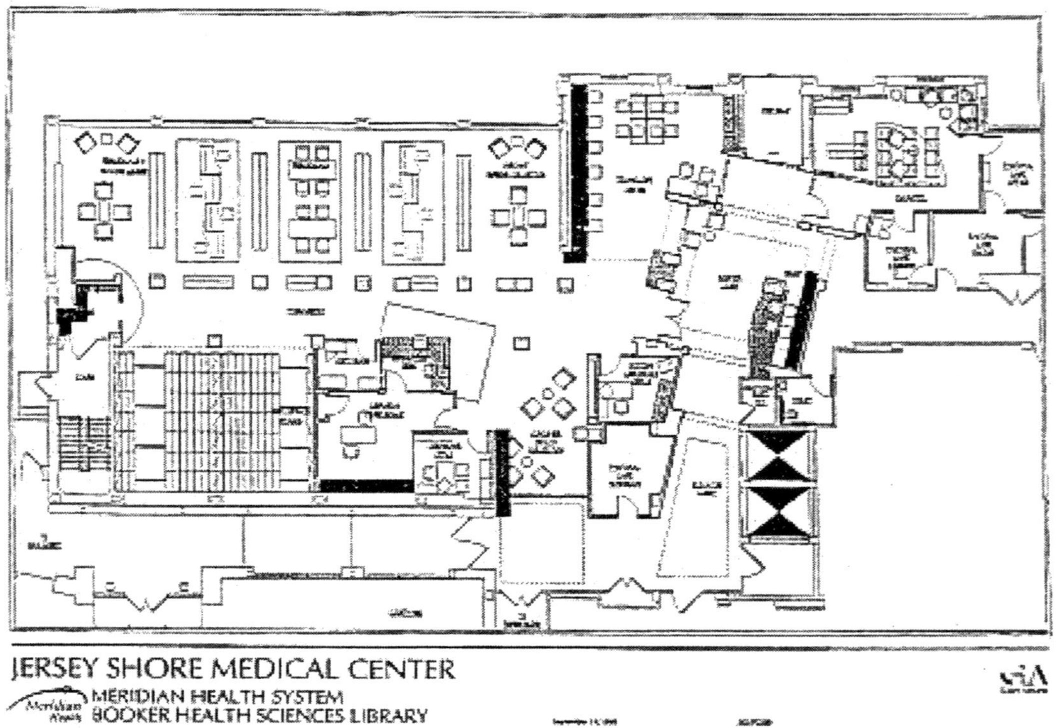

FIGURE 3.1. Booker Library floor plan. Drawn by Janet D. Megee. Reprinted with permission.

and label sets from MarciveWeb SELECT. Minimal monies were spent on the reclassification, and library staff had uninterrupted work time and control of the project.

During the same time period, construction began. Signs posted at the entrances to the Booker Pavilion announced the forthcoming health sciences library. An architectural rendering of the new library was displayed in the medical library. Periodically, articles were published in the Medical Center's weekly in-house newsletter to keep library customers informed about the construction project.

Without the knowledge of the library staff, the Medical Center started to renovate the building where the old School of Nursing was housed. Library staff discovered that the construction company working on the project would not protect the books and journals that were housed in the former nursing library as work was done on a new clinic area above. To protect the collection, library staff boxed the bound journals and sent them to an off-site storage facility until the new library was ready. The remaining book collection was boxed and stored in the hallway outside the medical library so the collection could be relabeled with the new call numbers prior to the move.

To ensure that the construction went as planned, the Vice President for Academic Affairs was involved with the weekly construction meetings. The library staff visited the construction site periodically to note its progress and to photograph the construction. In July, eleven new computers, approved on the capital budget process and purchased on a bulk capital order by the Information Technology department, arrived earlier than expected. Rather than storing the computers in Materials Management's receiving area, the library coordinator opted to install them in available carrel space in the medical library, a decision that was met with much appreciation from the library customers.

MOVING THE COLLECTIONS

The next challenge was the actual move. Library staff met with the moving company to learn how to prepare the collection for the move. To facilitate this preparation, the library stopped document delivery services for the months of December and January and changed its hours, opening for only three hours each morning during the last week of December and closing for the first two weeks in January. The move of the medical, nursing, stored nursing, and microfilm journal collections from four different locations proved to be the most challenging. On January 10, 2001, the move started and took less than three days to accomplish. The next week was spent reading the shelves and getting the library ready for business. Although it was not completely unpacked, the new Booker Health Sciences Library was opened and operational on January 22. The dream of a new library in the new millennium had finally come to pass (see Photos 3.1. and 3.2).

CONCLUSION

Everyone who visits the new library is amazed at its beauty and its functionality. The window-lined, cherrywood ambience is a radical change from the two former libraries. Features include areas for quiet study, leisure reading, and collaborative work. The Booker Health

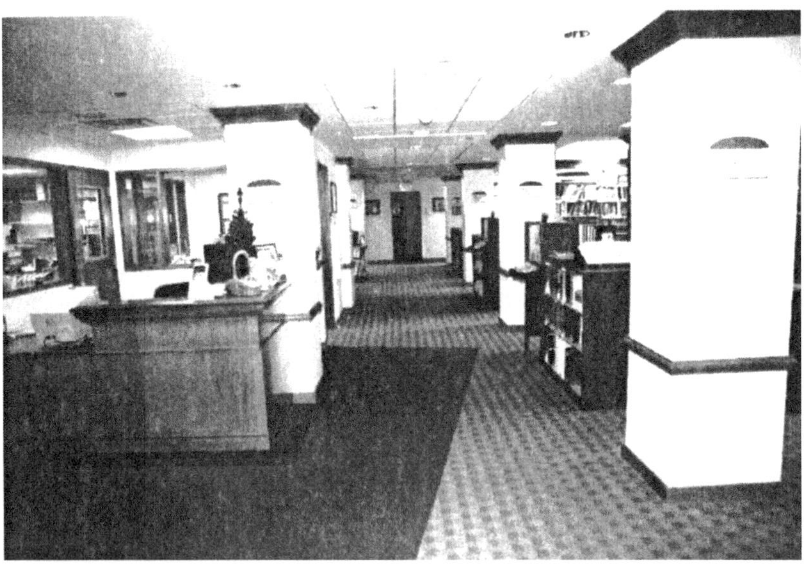

PHOTO 3.1. Booker Health Sciences Library. Photo by Chris Gahler. Reprinted with permission.

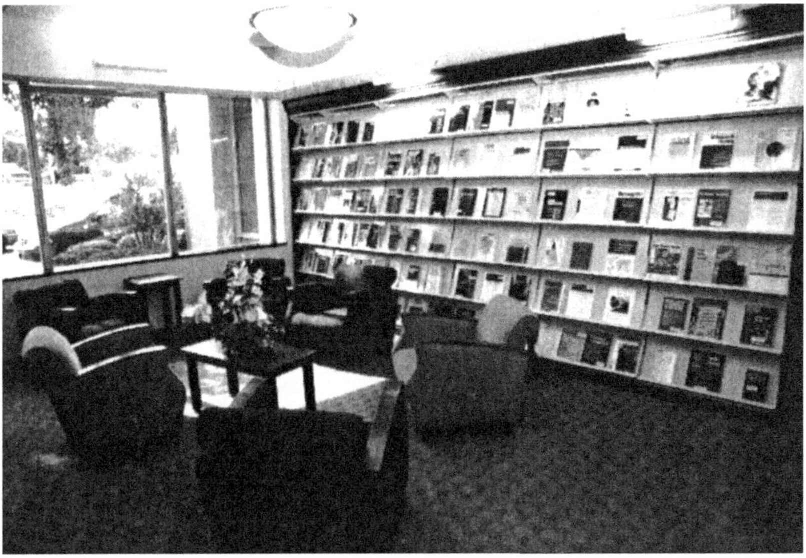

PHOTO 3.2. Ann May Nursing Collection. Photo by Chris Gahler. Reprinted with permission.

Sciences Library project brought together three distinct components of health care information (medicine, nursing, and consumer health) into a single, artistically beautiful facility that symbolizes the commitment by Meridian Health to health promotion, disease prevention, education, research, and clinical excellence.

NOTES

1. *Nursing Data Review 1997.* New York: National League for Nursing Press, 1997: 8.
2. Hitt, Samuel. "Administration: Space Planning for Health Sciences Libraries." In *Handbook of Medical Library Practice,* Fourth edition, edited by Louise Darling. Chicago: Medical Library Association, 1988: 387.
3. Ibid., p. 395.
4. Ibid., p. 397.

Case Study 4

A Tale of Two Libraries: Overview of a Merger

Elisabeth Jacobsen

OVERVIEW

Setting: Two city hospitals contracted to merge into a newly named 531-bed entity in January 2000. Although both had active libraries, the institutions differed widely. One was a Catholic, not-for-profit teaching hospital with an active residency program. The other was a public hospital with a long-standing nursing school. Despite these differences, only one hospital and one library would survive.

Objective: The project objective was to merge two equally sized libraries into one collection with half the space and half the manpower, while satisfying escalating demands for service.

Methods: First, an inventory was conducted of the journal and book collections of both libraries to identify duplications, tag inappropriate materials (outside the Catholic mission/directives), and to weed. Second, although one library was destined for closure, it still functioned within a working hospital that had informational needs. In the meantime, the libraries needed to embrace unity, even if only through a Web site. Finally, virtual presence provided access to collections, resources, and staff for those who did not have proximity to a physical library.

Results: The physical merger process took eighteen months longer than originally planned. The downside was that the library's physical move was chaotic because a nonlibrary mover was used, and reduction of staff levels caused hardship. The upside was that with one collection that was primarily microfilm based, and the other print, the journal collection acquired new depth and coverage without more space requirements. The book collection expanded considerably without expending budget funds because there was little duplication.

Conclusion: Considerable behind-the-scenes planning, inventories, flexibility, contingency planning, stamina, cooperation, and vision are required to ensure a successful merger.

INTRODUCTION

Established in 1879, Elizabeth General Medical Center featured 425 beds, and a School of Nursing dating back to 1891. St. Elizabeth Hospital, a 325-bed Catholic teaching hospital situated on the other side of the city, opened its doors in 1905 under the sponsorship of the Sisters of Charity of St. Elizabeth. Its thriving residency program had been in place for several decades.

Baptized with the new name Trinitas, the two hospitals had a new mission and a newly combined workforce. They faced the daunting task of creating a fresh, yet unified identity while phasing out one facility. In January 2000, Elizabeth General Medical Center and St. Elizabeth Hospital began the Herculean process of merging their missions and services. Both hospitals had long histories within the city, and unique identities, having coexisted for the better part of a century, serving those who lived and worked in or near the city of Elizabeth, New Jersey, deep in the heart of Union County.

PROJECT SUMMARY

After the paper merger, the end goal seemed simple: merge two libraries into one within six months or sooner. Achieving that goal was not simple because the project required planning, cooperation, communication, flexibility, creativity, and vision among players on all levels. Unexpected delays continually stalled the merger of library collections and services. From the beginning, the two biggest challenges for this consolidation project proved to be merging nearly equal-sized collections into half the space, with little, if any, downtime in library services during the move.

Both libraries held unique, extensive collections that reflected the needs of their respective institutions and programs. Collection duplications or overlap were minimal beyond core titles. To fulfill the needs of patrons from both institutions and anticipate needs of the new institution's future combined patronage, the challenge was planning ways to fit the collections of Library A (Elizabeth General) into the existing space of Library B (St. Elizabeth) without gaining any additional square footage.

Another challenge was meeting patron expectations that both libraries remain in service until just before consolidation, with minimal disruption to services, and availability of services in the new library in fewer than two weeks. Unfortunately, in the many months that followed, many unforeseen problems delayed the physical merger timeline, and added eighteen months to the original time frame.

Staffing

In the beginning phases of the merger, each library operated with one full-time library assistant. The director managed both libraries, and scheduled time between each location. As the merger drew closer to deadline, budgets were affected. Library A lost one position. Because that hospital was still operational, the director assumed the duties and ran a one-person library nearly full time. After a couple of months when it became evident that this approach was not working, Library A closed its doors, and all activities were shifted to Library B.

Early on, library staff learned that the merger process needed a fluid timeline since nearly every week brought changes and delays in the institutional master plan. Sometimes these delays worked to the library's advantage, affording sufficient time to conduct an intensive inventory of Library A and B's journal and monograph collections. This process helped identify duplications, flag materials from Library A's collection that were outside the Catholic doctrine and mission, and identify materials for weeding.

Collections

The fate of the monograph collections rested on several criteria: Brandon-Hill title lists, physician and faculty recommendations, edition, and institutional program needs since space was a priority consideration. Items were tagged with different color codes for instant identification during the various phases of the inventory process. Library A's reference and circulating items were integrated and Library B's collections were segregated. Also, Library B's nursing journals and monographs were arranged apart from the medical collections. The monographs were kept separate because of nursing student preference, but the journals were integrated back into the main archives. This created a more uniform flow of the collection, but required the shift of every title needed to create room for Library A's incoming titles.

The journal collections also proved to have little duplication apart from the core titles. The combined total of each library's preexisting collections exceeded 200 subscriptions. Since there would be zero growth in space allocation within the surviving library, deep cuts needed to be made. Plus, each institution's programs had a vested interest in the collections.

At journal renewal time, all duplicate titles were deleted from Library A's subscription list. The intention was to shift focus from Library A to Library B, making it the primary source of resources and services. For convenience, the list of deleted titles was posted in Library A. Since many of the deleted titles were core titles, the library tried to link to the corresponding full-text journal content whenever possible. If the title was not available online, the patron was instructed to request a copy of the article of interest from Library B. Document requests were then filled by fax or intercampus mail. One of the main advantages for deleting core titles was the cost savings. In 2001, fifty-eight duplicate titles were dropped at renewal, resulting in a savings of $13,500.

The libraries needed to create a new *combined journal holdings list* to reflect all changes. This list acted as a locator tool for the convenience of patrons and staff, in addition to creating a sense of unification. Each library displayed the new holdings lists at the reference desks of both libraries, and it was posted on the Web site as well.

Shelving

Shelving for monographs and archives was a critical issue. Library A had a compact shelving unit comprising the equivalent of forty-three bookcases with seven shelves each (301 shelves total) versus Library B's thirty-nine cases with five shelves each (195 shelves total) for a total loss of 106 shelves. Sixteen cases already housed the monograph collection in Library B. The rest of the shelf space was needed to hold journal backfiles, which comprised the bulk of the two collections. Bound and unbound backfiles older than five years had to be sacrificed. With few options for growth, alternative thinking was mandatory if the collections were to be successfully combined.

Archives

Inventories at both locations determined title runs and format. Library A's archives were a mixed batch of bound, unbound, and microfilm titles going back as far as twenty five years, the bulk of which was in microfilm format. Since very few title runs were duplicates, the microfilm collection offered a wealth of backfiles without taking up any more space. Library B's archives consisted of mostly unbound titles with a depth of around ten years for most titles.

Because space was at a premium, a decision was made to keep all duplicate titles in bound or microfilm format only, unless this was not an option. Each library's duplicate runs were also cross-referenced for the end purpose of building longer runs and filling gaps whenever possible. Once completed, Library B's archival collection would, at the very least, be tripled. Compared to what had existed separately, this was definitely the most positive benefit of the merger.

Equipment and Furnishings

Library A was well-furnished and decorated with paintings and silk plants in exotic pots. Furnishings included three computer stations, eight study carrels, comfortable lounge chairs, a coffee table, and an imposing reference desk. Library B, on the other hand, was more sparsely furnished. Its three computers were housed on a long conference table, with a cascade of tangled wires. This "computer hub" was placed inconveniently in the middle of the reference section between two small staff desks. No reference desk existed. Library B had no decorations other than a prominent cross.

Merging the collections was only a part of the challenge. Another hurdle was fitting existing furniture and squeezing three extra computers into Library B's new floor plan without losing too much seating. Whether or not the floor load could sustain the weight of the microfilm cabinets was a concern because years before, Library B's stacks were less than five-feet high instead of standard height because of this same concern.

In the end, no matter how it was all configured, seating space was cut. On the upside, several lovely paintings uplifted the ambience, and a comfortable reading nook was created from Library A's furniture stock. Unfortunately, the fate of the exotic planters and silk plants is still unknown, as they did not find their way over during the move.

Networking

Establishing vendor relationships are important in every business. Do not overlook potential advantages or perks that may come from this relationship. Over the years, familiarity can bring benefits, especially if the librarian carries the vendor over to a new institution, which was the case in this situation. Having had a positive past experience with consolidating collections at another institution, it made good business sense to reconnect with a vendor who was already an established contact.

For example, a microfilm vendor wanted unbound journals to fill gaps in his warehouse. The library needed microfilm to replace the titles being discarded because of lack of space and/or duplicate status. The library asked if journal backruns could be traded for microfilm credit, and this agreement provided a solution for shelf space problems and saved the library thousands of dollars. The only catch was that none of this could be done until just before the merger.

Services

Library services remained fully operational during all the phases of the merger. As mentioned, in the beginning stages the libraries remained status quo with separate staff. However, with two active hospitals, a residency program, nursing school, and a psychiatric facility all conducting business as usual, the demand for library services skyrocketed. Literature searches still needed to be performed for patient care or research papers, and document delivery requests needed to be processed. Between both libraries over 4,500 interlibrary loans were processed, and over 525 literature searches were performed during that first year of transition.

The Virtual Library

The decision to shut down one library was not without protest. In terms of library services, it was imperative that the patrons of Library A not feel abandoned. Fortunately, since everything was in flux, and being redesigned, it was the perfect time to latch on to new technology to create organization out of chaos.

As they say, timing is everything. With the birth of a new hospital also came a new Web site. This was the window of opportunity for the library to reach out to all its customers who no longer had a physical library, and provide outreach to those at the psychiatric facility without library services at all. Although very few departments at either hospital had representation or active pages on the Web site, it did not take much to plead the case for the library to develop a site.

Equipped with a Web presence, the library could now redefine itself virtually and physically. There was some resistance at first. Many library customers needed guidance, as well as reassurance that the "virtual library" could satisfy many of their needs until the libraries were totally merged.

The first version of the library's Web site offered little more than the basics: e-mail access to the library staff, hours of operation, phone numbers, mission statement, etc. This was to done merely as a first step to establish the library's presence as a link on the hospital's main Web site. In the ensuing months, the Web site evolved and became more functional, offering links to full-text databases, reference resources, and information on program-specific subject areas, such as nursing and others. Later, literature search and document delivery e-forms were posted on the Web site for the added convenience of the library's customers.

Having a Web site and having customers aware of it are two different things. Publicizing the Web site was a critical component for success. Aside from the usual posters and flyers distributed and posted throughout the hospitals, more was needed. Over the next eighteen months, the Public Relations department promoted the library's Web site in the hospital newsletters many times. In addition, a PowerPoint presentation given at a monthly multicampus directors' meeting provided an overview and introduction to the Web site's features and functions.

There was a learning and acceptance curve. Traditional library users balked at first; many users were not computer savvy, still others missed having the library as a physical entity, but eventually they all adapted. Born out of necessity for survival several years ago, the Web site today is now an integral library resource with high-volume usage. The current students and residents can no more fathom the library without its electronic arm of resources than could the users of yesterday imagine being without *Index Medicus.*

PROJECT TIMELINE

There was an unexpected eighteen months between preparation for the merger and the actual move. These delays brought both benefits and frustrations. On one hand, the delays allowed the library time to prepare and create new resource pathways. On the downside, the delays often frazzled the patrons, the staff, and strained the budget.

January 2000: The merger begins: both hospitals acquire a new name, and are "one."

January 2001: A year later, the growing pains are evident. The hospitals still have two of nearly everything, and for the most part, run things separately. Each library still has separate budgets, journal subscriptions, and staff. From a fiscal perspective the subscription accounts cannot be merged into one working list at renewal time because both budgets remain divided.

March 2001: The "Microfilm Exchange Project" was now underway. As a result, the library gained fifty-five rolls of free microfilm, plus hundreds of dollars of additional purchase credit from the microfilm vendor. The "physicians only" after-hours access policy was expanded to meet the needs of the floor nurses, residents, medical students, and nursing students. E-mail access to the library staff was activated on the library's Web site, as was the new, unified holdings list. Forty-eight online journal links were added to the Web site, plus twelve full-text databases.

May 2001: The library director designs a preliminary floor plan. Furniture from Library A will be used as a cost-saving measure. For the first time, office space for the director was mentioned. The move was rescheduled for August 2001. Library A will close for on-site business in June 2001. All patrons were urged to use the Web site. Library A ceases filling interlibrary loan requests from outside institutions. All document delivery and search requests are processed through Library B.

June 2001: The library is suddenly given a new location in the basement. An alternate floor plan quickly is designed. The new location is even smaller than either of the currently existing libraries. Due to financial constraints, the recommendation to use a specialized library moving company is overruled in favor of using the hospital's commercial mover.

July 2001: Consultants determine that the basement location will be unsuitable, and the project is back to the original plan. The floor load bearing ability of Library B becomes a concern. More consultants measure Library B and create a floor plan for furniture, equipment, and staff areas. Due to lack of space, not all furniture can be incorporated into Library B. Five study carrels have to be sacrificed. In exchange, Library B will lose two study tables and seating. Access to the library was restricted to physicians or nurses for research related to patient care only. Library A's technician position was eliminated. The library staff now consists of the director and an assistant. The end of July is announced as the scheduled move.

August 2001: Library move postponed.

September 2001: A rescheduled move date is not on the institutional calendar. Without staff at Library A, it is now impossible to service any customers or fill any loans from the collection. Library A's journal collection is designated "lost" for the time being. Journal subscriptions are finally merged into one account for 2002. The library's move date is still uncertain, everything comes to a halt as nothing more can be done. The shelves in Library B are over 75 percent full. More drastic cuts need to be done prior to the physical move. Lack of available dumpsters impedes progress, sometimes for days. September 11 events impact everyone on every level of operation, most especially due to the close proximity to New York City, causing even more delays.

November 2001: The move.

ISSUES AND PROBLEMS

Several issues and problems affected the project. The commercial movers were not prepared to move a library collection by chronological, alphabetical, or classification order and needed constant supervision. The color-coded tagging system so carefully devised proved pointless. Even worse, since there were only two library staff members, one person needed to be in each library supervising. The furniture from Library A did not fit. A spontaneous, redesigned floor plan had to be created on the spot. As a result of consultant error, two carrels were unable to fit the floor plan, causing a loss of two computer stations. Construction for the director's office was initiated, and then halted for several weeks without explanation or a timeline for completion. This affected the reference area since three bookcases were emptied to accommodate construction equipment. It took nearly two months to complete this construction. An unexpected surprise was that the engineering design did not include connections to heating or air-conditioning ducts. The movers left more than 220 large, four-foot-long boxes stacked three deep upon each another *in no logical order.* The boxes lined the hospital hallway from one end to the other and spilled over into the library. Even worse, half the boxes had no identifying tags or labels. Boxes that were labeled were usually buried several boxes under the mystery boxes. Patrons expected library services to continue without interruption.

LESSONS LEARNED

To avoid some of the problems encountered in this project, a number of lessons were learned that could benefit others, including the following:

- Insist on contracting a mover specializing in libraries. Although the institution may think it is saving up-front costs by using a commercial moving company, in the long run it is neither time nor cost-effective if the staff has to do damage control at the other end.
- Request additional help. Educate upper management about the reality of moving and shifting heavy books, even if it means

handing a huge book or box of books to a decision maker to prove this point.

- Become a control freak. In an ideal world it would be nice if library staff could rely on everyone's expertise. Measure everything yourself, not once but many times. Get an industrial tape measure and keep it ready at all times. Question floor plans created by "designers," especially if they seem to fit everything you could not fit in your own design! Do not expect anyone to take accountability if the floor plan does not work. The last thing you want to hear on moving day is, "This will not fit. Now what?"
- Befriend the facilities and housekeeping staff. Sometimes they can pull strings for you that no amount of huffing and puffing will get.
- Bring candy and small snacks as a token "thank-you" to the hospital departments that help with the move, and customers when times get tough and frustrating. In addition, a smile and sense of humor work wonders.
- Set limits. Some patrons will do anything to continue using the library. In this project, without limits enforced with an iron hand, there was no deterring those who felt entitled to use the library anytime, under any conditions, even during construction, moving, and unpacking.
- Do not mistake patrons covertly unpacking and digging in boxes as a sign they are volunteering to help.
- Be realistic about the project. If you think it will take two weeks to do it all, multiply that estimate by two. Give yourself more time for downtime, not less. If you manage to get it all done in less time, people will be impressed. If you give yourself a tight timeframe and need more time, people will grumble and wonder what is "taking so long?"

CONCLUSION

A successful merger will involve myriad planning stages. Be prepared to wear multiple hats and expend a lot of energy with behind-the-scenes preparations. Every detail, from inventories, to floor plans, customer service issues, shifting, down to the location of electrical outlets must be addressed in the action plan. It is equally important to create contingency plans, because things can and will go wrong. Still, the most important ingredients for success are flexibility, vision, and never losing sight of the end goal because although you may not be creating a whole new universe, this challenge comes pretty close.

SUGGESTED READING

Library Space Planning Guide. Hartford, CT: Connecticut State Library, 2002. Available online at <http://www.cslib.org/libbuild.htm>.

The Medical Library Association Guide to Managing Health Care Libraries. Edited by Ruth Holst and Sharon A. Phillips. New York: Neal-Schuman Publishers, 2000.

Planning Library Facilities. Bloomington: Illinois Wesleyan University, Medical Library Association, 1993.

Space Planning in the Special Library. Washington, DC: Special Libraries Association, 1991.

Case Study 5

Renovating a Small Hospital Library

Veronica Dawn Stewart

OVERVIEW

Setting: The Saint Francis Health Sciences Library serves the physicians, nurses, and support staff of the Saint Francis Health System. The health system consists of two general hospitals, one psychiatric hospital, and a physicians' clinic with locations throughout northeastern Oklahoma. Located on the ground level of Saint Francis Hospital, the health system's flagship location, the library houses more than 100 current print journals, 1,200 books, open-access computers, and three full-time employees within a space of 1,500 square feet. The library also shares space with the Pharmacy's Drug Information Center.

Objectives: The objectives for the remodeling included giving the medical librarian an office; increasing the number of open-access computers; creating a less cumbersome traffic flow; and updating the look of the space.

Methods: The remodeling project was in the planning stages for six years before the money was appropriated and a timetable was established. Three library staff members packed all the books and journals with assistance from three hospital volunteers. The materials and furnishings were stored in a trailer parked at one of the hospital's receiving docks for the duration of the project. Since the library had to remain open during the remodeling and the storage trailer could not hold all the library materials and furnishings at once, the process took place in two stages. The stacks and public-access computer area were packed, gutted, and remodeled first, followed by the library and Drug Information staff areas. All staff remained in the library during the entire remodeling process.

Results/conclusions: All project objectives were achieved within a timely manner and with very few complications. Future revisions may be needed as the collection grows and patron needs change, but the renovated library now has a more pleasing and less-institutional appearance.

INTRODUCTION

Setting

The Saint Francis Health Sciences Library serves the physicians, nurses, and support staff of the Saint Francis Health System of Tulsa, Oklahoma. The health system encompasses more than 800 staffed beds contained at two general hospitals, Saint Francis Hospital and Saint Francis Hospital at Broken Arrow, and one psychiatric facility, Laureate Psychiatric Clinic and Hospital. The health system employs nearly 900 physicians at these hospitals and affiliated clinics located throughout northeastern Oklahoma.

The Saint Francis Health Sciences Library is housed in a 1,500 square-foot space on the ground floor of Saint Francis Hospital. Library staff consists of two professional librarians and one library assistant. The library also houses the Pharmacy's Drug Information Center. The library office space includes a small kitchen and storage room.

History

The library was established in the 1960s by Dr. Robert Tompkins, who was medical director of the hospital at the time. Initially located in the hospital's basement, the library soon moved to the first floor near the physicians' entrance and lounge. During nearly two decades in this location, the library grew from a staff of one managing a few donated materials into an active department that is a highly visible and integral part of the hospital.

In 1991, when space usage on the main floor of the hospital changed, the library was moved one level down to the ground floor of the hospital. This location was the only room available at the time. The space was L-shaped and had originally been designed for use as the outpatient pharmacy. Although this location was not as visible to the physicians, it was in a high traffic area since it was on the same floor as the cafeteria. It was also convenient for the Drug Information staff as the central pharmacy is also on the same floor (see Figure 5.1).

The library features a collection of 1,200 books and 100 current print journal subscriptions as well as a small collection of audio- and videotapes. The library does not own or support multimedia items such as CD-ROMs, DVDs, or microforms. The library's online resources include more than 800 journals, nearly 100 books, and more than 30 electronic databases. All of the library's online resources are accessible throughout the health system-wide intranet.

Objectives

The push for remodeling the space began almost as soon at the library was settled into its current location. Minor changes were made such as replacing a display window with a book drop, but the decor remained institutional with beige walls, gray carpet, and abstract art that was uniform with other artwork in the hospital. Not long after Beth Treaster, the current medical librarian, joined the staff in 1996, she began to petition the hospital administration and the library committee for funding to completely remodel the space. At first, the project was intended to be a facelift, but as the library expanded its services, collection, and personnel, the need for more extensive changes became evident (see Photo 5.1).

Approval Process

Saint Francis Health System has a detailed plan for the submission of renovation plans, and approval for funding is the primary concern. As part of the application process, the medical librarian stated roughly what was needed in the library and consulted the hospital engineering department about the approximate costs. The resulting figure was then submitted for approval.

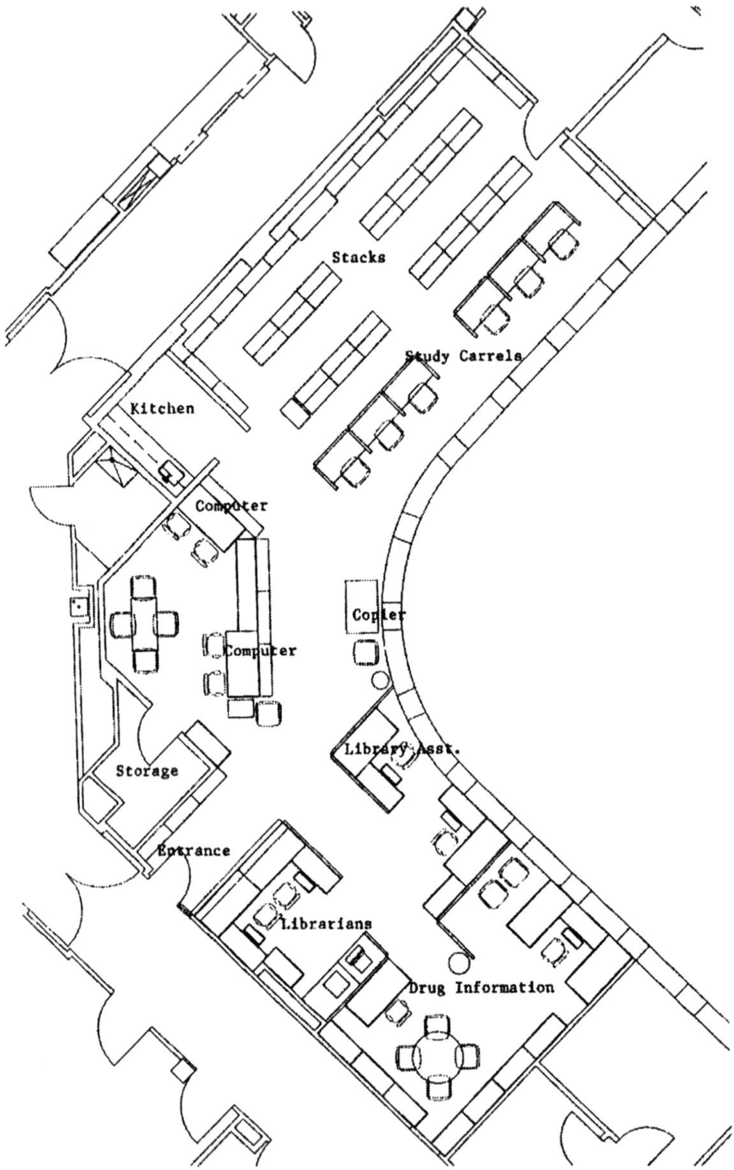

FIGURE 5.1. Layout before remodeling. Drawing by Dennis Linscheid. Reprinted with permission.

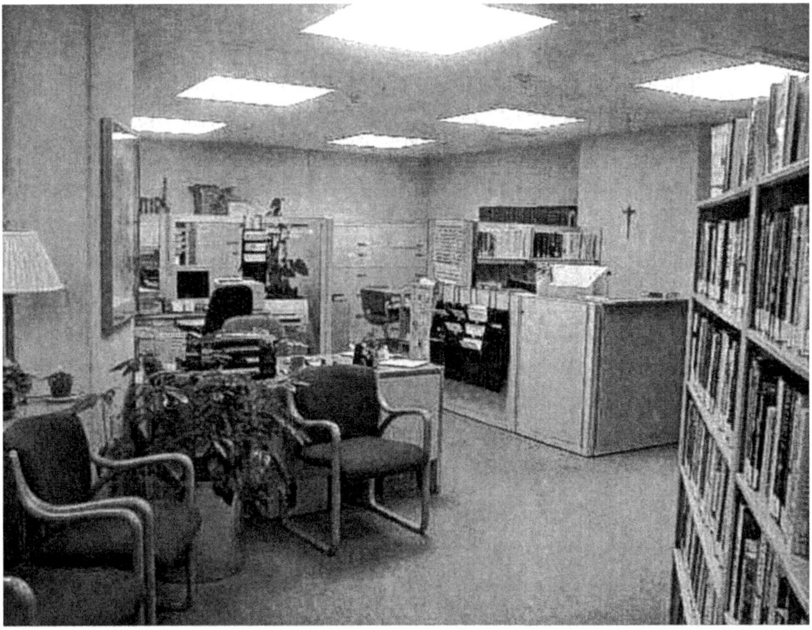

PHOTO 5.1. Staff area before remodeling. Photo by Jacyntha Sterling. Reprinted with permission.

Renovation Goals

Although the hospital administration and library committee members were in agreement that the library needed to be freshened up, revenue-generating departments take precedence in the renovation approval process. As a result, the medical librarian applied for renovation funding six years before the request was approved and the project was scheduled. Although the needs of the staff and patrons continually evolved, the basic goals of the renovation remained relatively unchanged throughout this process and included the following:

- Build an office for the medical librarian.
- Increase the number of open-access computers.
- Create a cleaner traffic flow.
- Update the look of the space.

Staff

When the library staff was increased to three persons in 2002, the librarian needed private office space. Prior to this, the medical librarian and the library assistant sat behind a counter beside the front door. This left them out in the open, making it easy for patrons to consult them. But the librarian lacked a place for private meetings. When the assistant librarian was hired, she took the place of the library assistant behind the counter, the library assistant moved to a separate desk, and the medical librarian took the place of the assistant librarian's desk. That same year, the Drug Information Center staff was increased by three, with the addition of a resident, leaving their department secretary seated out in the library. Space for this department needed to be increased and the furnishings rearranged so the secretary might move back into the Drug Information space.

Computers

The library has a history of making computers available to the Saint Francis staff at-large and the medical librarian was determined to continue that tradition and increase the number of open-access computers. Although computers are available throughout the hospital, not all staff members have access to them. The library computers are available to all Saint Francis staff members, residents, and students as well as patient family members for research, education, and in the case of patient family members, e-mail.

In 1996, the first open-access computer was installed and featured word processing and a modem for dial-up access to the Internet. By 2001 a separate printer and four computers equipped with Microsoft Office programs and a T-1 Internet connection were set up for open use. These computers were placed on standard office tables, which offered little privacy or workspace. During the school year frequent use by residents, nursing, and pharmacy students left many people waiting for a turn or just turning around and walking out the door. The medical librarian wished to increase the computers to six and to change the physical arrangement to provide more privacy and workspace to those who needed it.

Layout

Over the years the available open space for traffic flow and movement around the library had been chiseled away as staff and resources were added, and the arrangement of these additions was not always optimal. This led to cumbersome layouts in the two most important areas of the library: the entryway and the open-access computer area.

The library's sole entrance door was hazardous. It was defined by the counter, behind which the medical librarian and assistant librarian sat. The door opened back to the storage room wall. Although the single entrance made the area easy to secure, the immediate availability of library personnel sometimes resulted in patrons getting hit by the door as others tried to enter. Although neither the wall nor the counter could be moved, rearranging the staff and installing a glass barrier to discourage patrons from stopping just inside the door would reduce the potential for near catastrophes.

The arrangement of the open-access computers also contributed to problems of traffic flow. The four computers were arranged in a line, two per table, with the printer placed on a media cabinet between the two tables. Since there was not enough space to extend the computers in a straight line, the whole area slanted outward and formed an obtuse angle. A study table on the inside of the angle further cluttered this clumsy arrangement. Shelving added to the outside of the tables left a narrow opening just wide enough for one person to pass between the computers and outside wall to reach the study carrels and stack area of the library. The computer arrangement had to be straightened out and the computers redistributed to make the stack area more visible and easier to access.

Color Scheme

Once the project was approved, the most agonizing part of planning was choosing the colors for the library's new paint and wallpaper. The medical librarian toured other areas of the hospital that had been recently remodeled and consulted the staff of both the library and Drug Information departments to see what was available and to get ideas. In the end, the engineering department suggested a paint and carpet combination of off-white walls and maroon variegated carpet with accenting wallpaper borders that was approved by all consulted.

Project Exclusions

The remodeling goals clearly defined areas that the project would address and not address. Demolition, building, and expansion were not part of the project. Although the medical librarian did briefly consider expanding the workroom to serve as her office, this idea was quickly abandoned when engineers discovered that one of the walls could not be moved because it was a main structural wall. Expansion of the library into surrounding space also was not an option as the spaces that border the library were occupied and there were no plans for their vacancy.

The library's odd shape did have one advantage—other than the workroom wall, the space was free of columns and support beams. Shelves and furnishings could be placed without concern or obstructions. Portable walls would be used to define the medical librarian's office space and Drug Information departments.

In lieu of purchasing new furnishings, a desk for the Ariel terminal and a table for the typewriter were salvaged from the hospital's surplus furniture stores. The medical librarian also arranged to have several chairs recovered so they would match, and instead of purchasing a worktable to stand beside the copier, a book cart was repainted. New artwork was selected from the hospital surplus and a decorative map was purchased. Ancient curtains that were removed for painting simply were not replaced.

METHODS

Planning for the care of the collection and staff during the remodeling proved to be as large a project as planning for the remodeling itself. The hospital contracted with a company for assistance in the moving and storage of furniture and materials, but the work of packing and organizing these items fell on the library staff. The assistant librarian searched the library literature for information on managing a collection and keeping services available during a renovation project. Although it was not possible to hire professional library movers, ideas for evaluating the collection and labeling and numbering materials for quick return to the shelves were useful.[1-3]

PREPARATION

A few weeks before packing was scheduled to start, the medical librarian weeded the collection. A few journal titles were completely removed from the collection and made available to other libraries through the Backmed Listserv (<http://lists.swetsblackwell.com/mailman/listinfo/backmed>). Most of the books culled from the circulating collection, along with books that had been donated to the library but not added to the collection, went into a book sale. The sale was a one-day event held in a meeting room just outside the cafeteria, guaranteeing high traffic. Funds from the book sale were used to purchase new materials.

SHELVING GAINS

A larger concern in weeding was finding a new home for the library's historical collection. The collection had been donated to the library by its founder, Dr. Tompkins, with the stipulation that the items were never to be used. The early texts, including a volume of *History of Magic and Experimental Science* by Lynn Thorndike and a complete set of *The Collected Essays of Sir William Osler* were kept in a locked cabinet in the middle of the bound journals. The cabinet looked impressive but took up space that was needed for journal shelving. With the consent of the donor's family, arrangements were made to donate the collection to the History of Medicine Collection of the Robert M. Bird Health Sciences Library at the University of Oklahoma Health Sciences Center, where the items would be reunited with the rest of Dr. Tompkins' papers. The cabinet itself, which was not part of the donation to the Saint Francis Library, was given to the hospital's legal department.

Additional shelving was also gained by reducing the amount of space allotted to current journal display. In previous years the library used both sides of an entire line of shelving to display new journal issues. At the end of 2002, due to the increasing availability of online journals, dozens of print journal subscriptions were dropped. This left the library with more new journal display space than was needed, so the space was reduced by half. The outside of the shelves would remain for the display of new journals, but the backside was converted to standard shelving for the circulating books. Substantial amounts of the donated nonmedical books were weeded, freeing up additional space. This allowed the nursing collection to be moved from the back of the library where it had been overflowing its shelves, to the more prominent location in the middle of the library (see Photo 5.2).

No environmental concerns existed and remodeling would rectify the one safety concern. Although the library had off-site storage that was used for older journals, the library still did not have enough shelf space for all the journal backfiles, so some items were placed on top of the shelves. The librarian had gotten permission from the hospital to do this, but the safety inspectors occasionally took note of this practice. The journal collection weeding and additional shelving eliminated the need to place items on top of the shelves.

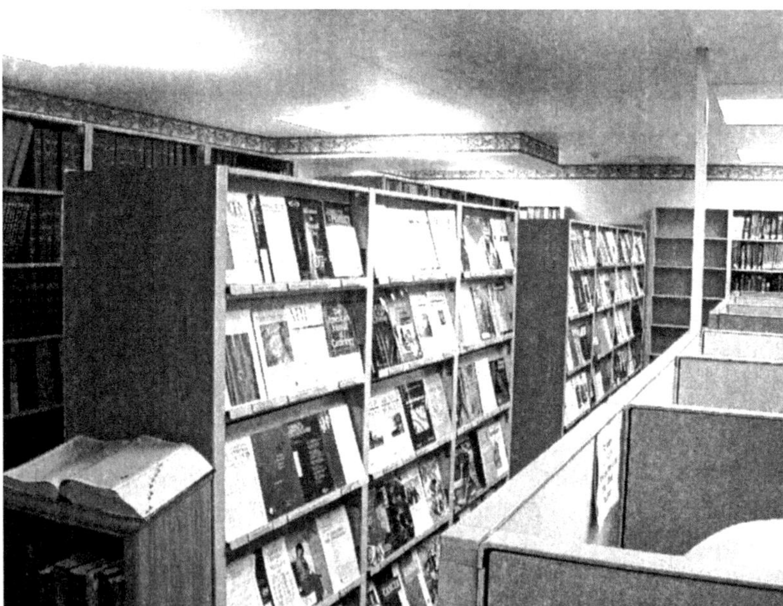

PHOTO 5.2. Remodeled new journal display area. Photo by Randy Kindy. Reprinted with permission.

MAINTAINING PATRON SERVICE

To publicize the fact that the library would be accessible during the renovations, hospital personnel were notified with a message on the front page of the library Web site and a sign on the library door. Since the print collection would be inaccessible for approximately four weeks, the library was placed on inactive status on DOCLINE. Orders for articles could still be placed and announcements to hospital staff stressed that anything that was unattainable from the library collection during this time could be ordered.

Although closing the library would have allowed the staff and volunteers to focus solely on packing and preparations for remodeling, the medical librarian felt that it would be a disservice to the hospital at large.[4] Not only did the library remain open and accessible throughout the remodeling process, but the library staff also remained within the library itself. Given the library's unorthodox space, the engineering department had planned a two-stage remodeling process. The stack and open-access computer areas were gutted and remodeled first, followed by the staff area. This plan actually helped accomplish the goal of keeping the library open and staffed throughout the remodeling.

The library staff and volunteers began packing the book and journal collections two weeks before the remodeling crews were due to arrive. An article by Myers suggested the use of actual library movers who could provide special book trucks designed to move and store the contents of entire shelves.[5] The moving company hired by the hospital did not specialize in libraries, but the movers provided five large all-purpose trucks that were perfect for books and journals. The trucks held the entire book collection and one-fifth of the journal collection, leaving the remainder to be packed in boxes.

To keep the boxes and trucks straight the assistant librarian devised a labeling system. Although the collection would be shifted during its return to the shelves, labeling would ensure that the items were unpacked in the same order as they were packed. All the shelves were labeled as a simple grid with each section numbered and each shelf lettered. Items removed from a shelf and placed into a box or truck were labeled with the shelf section number and shelf letter from which they were removed.

The movers stored items and furnishings from the library in a trailer parked at one of the hospital loading docks for the duration of the remodeling. They also did the physical work of breaking down shelves and furnishings. Most open-access and staff computers were disconnected and stored by the hospital's Information Technology department.

The library and Drug Information staff remained in the library and worked within the space that was not under renovation at the time. Computer access was limited during the time that each section was under renovation, but the library assistant's computer was kept on-site at all times for DOCLINE access. A plastic curtain protected the staff from the sanding and painting, but the noise, dust, and fumes still drifted into the staff area. The entire library was unpleasant and patrons largely stayed away once the renovators arrived to do their jobs.

RESULTS

When the remodeling crews left and the furnishings and materials were completely restored six weeks later, the major goals of the remodeling project were satisfactorily completed. The medical librarian's office was large enough for an L-shaped desk, credenza, and an extra chair for a guest. The number of public-access computers was increased from four to six, with three of the computers situated in study carrels that had been rarely used by library patrons. The new computer arrangement and subsequent adjustment of the shelves opened up the pathway leading back to the stack area. Weeding of the book collection allowed library staff to leave the bottom shelves and an entire section of shelves vacant and available for future acquisitions. Finally, the new maroon carpet and off-white walls set the library apart from the gray and beige hallways outside the door (see Photo 5.3).

ABANDONED IDEAS AND PLANS GONE AWRY

Although the major goals of the remodeling were achieved, a few smaller goals were discarded early in the planning stages. In the original plans, workspace for the library volunteers and an area for comfortable reading chairs were planned. But, there simply was not enough room within the library for these areas.

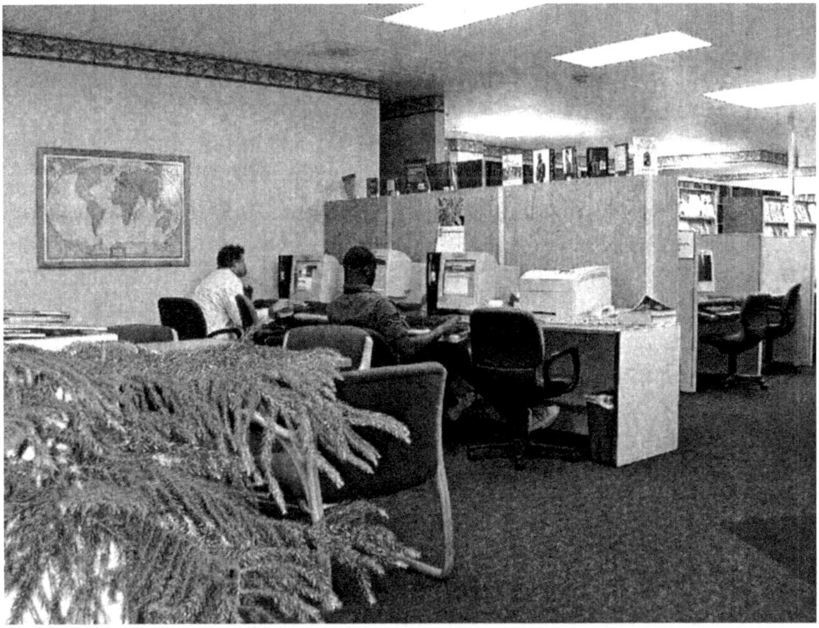

PHOTO 5.3. Patrons at the new open-access computer area. Photo by Randy Kindy. Reprinted with permission.

As with any project, not all went as planned. In an effort to return materials to the shelves quickly, library staff and hospital volunteers began unpacking journals from both the beginning and the end of the alphabet at the same time, hoping to meet somewhere in the middle. Believing that weeding and the additional shelving would result in extra space in the journal shelving area, space was left between titles for additional items, but the staff overestimated the amount of space that was gained. The end result was that the reshelving met in the middle with a substantial number of journals still in boxes. All shelved journals had to be shifted in order to fit in the remaining journals, which delayed the return of some items to the shelves.

CONCLUSION

After the painters and carpet layers left, patrons who had been scarce during the remodeling returned to find an updated and pleasant space. An article on the renovation was published in the physician newsletter and an announcement was placed on the library Web site. All hospital staff were notified that the project was over and invited to stop by and take a tour.

No adjustments have been made to the original plan, but future changes are planned. One little-used journal has already returned to its place on top of the shelves and the journal collection will have to be shifted again following the first bindery delivery in 2004. Ideas under consideration include shifting the books to make the reference collection more visible or completely eliminating the separate reference collection, as more books become available online. The non-medical collection will be further reduced as the books age, thus making more space available for medical texts and journals. Compared to the drama of renovation, these are minor adjustments any vibrant, useful library must constantly make.

NOTES

1. Myers, Charles. "A Mover That Only Moves Libraries." *American Libraries* 23(April 1992): 332-333.

2. Grey, Billie J. "Making Your Move." *American Libraries* 23(April 1992): 330-331.

3. Stout, Betty. "Managing a Move, Without a Hitch." *Book Report* 15(January/February 1997): 27-29.

4. Moreland, Virginia F., Robison, Carolyn L., and Stephens, Joan M. "Moving a Library Collection: Impact on Staff Morale." *Journal of Academic Librarianship* 19(March 1993): 8-11.

5. Myers, "A Mover That Only Moves Libraries," p. 332.

Case Study 6

Blending the New with the Old: Designing a New Library in a Historic Naval Hospital

Jane A. Pellegrino
Lisa R. Eblen

OVERVIEW

Setting: The Library Services Department of the Naval Medical Center Portsmouth (NMCP) serves the Command's 5,000 staff members, patients, and family members. The Command includes a 286-bed hospital and extensive outpatient clinics. NMCP is one of three major teaching hospitals in the Navy.

Objective: In the new facility, the planners sought to create a library with state-of-the-art technology that demonstrated the Command's commitment to learning.

Methods: Planning for the new library facility began with plans for the construction of a new acute care facility. In 1995 the staff of the library began working closely with the Health Facilities Planning and Project Office (HFPPO) to review the original architect's drawings and make recommendations for revisions. Although planning was constrained by the structural walls of the 1830 building, collaboration among the library

The authors would like to acknowledge the following individuals for their invaluable contributions to the renovation of the Library: Suad Jones, MLS, AHIP, Head Medical Librarian, Naval Medical Center Portsmouth, 1977-2001; Alfred J. Ciuizo, LCDR, MSC, USN (Ret.), Health Facilities Planning and Project Office; Robert C. Vogler, CDR, NC, USN, Health Facilities Planning and Project Office; and Deborah A. Mortland, LCDR, MSC, USN, Health Facilities Planning and Project Office.

staff, HFPPO, architects, interior designers, and shelving experts produced an excellent design.

Results: In August 2002, NMCP Library Services moved to a new library in the recently renovated Naval Hospital. In the move from a cramped 3,200 square-foot space into a spacious 14,000 square-foot facility, the health sciences and general libraries were integrated for the first time. The new facility provides space for the library collections, staff offices, studying and meeting areas, and has attracted new clientele. The nineteenth-century architecture, views of the Elizabeth River, and state-of-the-art networking and public access computers invite the staff. The swipecard system allows 24/7 access for NMCP staff.

Conclusions: Close attention to detail and ongoing modifications within budget guidelines were essential to success. A commodious atmosphere and state-of-the-art equipment draw patrons. Although it is said that form should follow function, library functions can be fit into existing space with imagination and an eye for design.

INTRODUCTION

The Library Services Department at NMCP provides professional and general library services through its Health Sciences Library and Crew's Library. On October 1, 2002, Library Services started the new fiscal year by hosting an open house that officially welcomed the staff of Naval Medical Center Portsmouth to a new, expanded facility in the recently renovated 1830 Naval Hospital building. For the first time the medical and general library collections were combined. The new library facility has a "Barnes & Noble" atmosphere with state-of-the-art networking and computer capabilities. The nineteenth-century architecture and the views of the Elizabeth River and the cities of Portsmouth and Norfolk invite the staff to work or relax apart from their busy workspaces.

Setting

NMCP serves the medical needs of the half-million military beneficiaries in the Tidewater, Virginia, area. NMCP includes three main buildings on its Portsmouth campus and nine branch medical clinics. Charette Health Care Center (CHCC), the main clinical facility, is a modern 286-bed hospital with extensive outpatient clinics. Building 215, the hospital that now serves as office and clinical space, flanks CHCC on one side. The original hospital, Building 1, is on the other side. NMCP is one of three major teaching hospitals in the Navy. Its extensive graduate medical education program includes internships and residency training in thirteen specialty areas.

The Library

The Library Services Department is comprised of three librarians and two library technicians, and serves a Command of 5,500 military and civilian personnel and the patients and family members of NMCP. Since 2002, medical and general collections and services have been under a single management. The Health Sciences Library offers an extensive print and online collection, interlibrary loan, and reference service. The Crew's Library offers recreational reading materials and services similar to those found in a public library. Library Services includes a special collection within the library, known as the Patient and Family Resource Center, offering lay health materials for patients and their families. Patients and family members are also welcome to use the computers or look for health information or leisure reading materials.

The Health Sciences Library offers current print and online books, over 500 scholarly journal subscriptions in print, and approximately 400 online journals. Library Services supports patient care, graduate medical education, research, continuing education, and undergraduate and graduate programs of Navy College. Resources provided by the Telelibrary Project of the Bureau of Medicine and Surgery and the Navy General Library Program supplement the Command's resources. The library also provides a meeting place for collaborative work. Its resources are delivered to the point of care through its Web site and telephone and e-mail reference services.

Historically, the general and professional libraries at NMCP were separate. A description of the original hospital mentions that "next to the mess hall was a space known as the 'Smoking Room,' which served as the first 'Library.'"[1] When the hospital was renovated and expanded following the Spanish-American War, the number of inpatients increased and activities expanded. The first recreational library was established in a small room on the third floor of Building 1. In 1919, the American Library Association assigned a librarian to the hospital who "added a great deal to the comfort and happiness of the patients."[2] When the Association stopped this support, the librarian became an employee of the Navy. The recreational library had several base locations during its history, moving first to Building 1 and then to Building 215.

In 1945, residency programs were established in general surgery and obstetrics/gynecology, and by 1948 there were ten internship programs based at the Naval Hospital. The Medical Library was established in Building 1 to provide professional library services and remained there until 1960 when it moved to the second floor of Building 215, the new clinical facility. In the decades that followed, the Medical Library built extensive journal and book collections and a reputation for excellent service (see Photo 6.1).

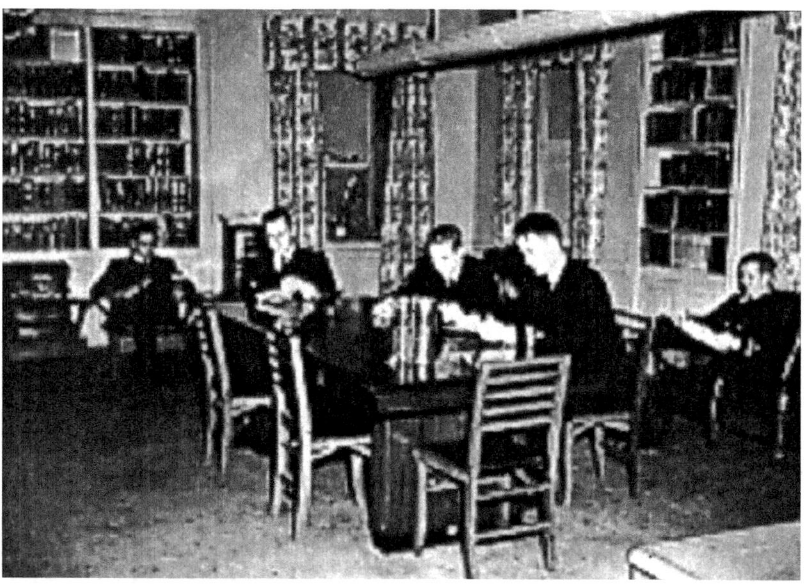

PHOTO 6.1. Medical officers in the Medical Library in the 1950s. Official U.S. Navy photo.

Over the years the Medical and Crew's Libraries developed in parallel, each serving a different clientele. Space constraints caused the closure of the Crew's Library in 1994. The following year, the head medical librarian proposed the realignment of the libraries under one management in the renovated Building 1. The proposal was approved and plans for the combined facility began. As part of the Command realignment that took place in 2001, the Medical Library became the Health Sciences Library.

The Building

Naval Hospital, Portsmouth, is the oldest continuously running hospital in the Navy. Construction of the first Naval hospital began on the site of the former Fort Nelson in 1827 and the hospital opened for patient care in July 1830. The four-story building is a granite structure built around a courtyard. The open end was originally bridged by a wooden structure, which has since been replaced. The building's entire front was faced with chisel-dressed Virginia freestone, with a portico of ten Doric columns fronted by twenty steps that are ninety-two feet wide. The hospital is known as Building 1. During its long history the Naval Hospital has undergone several major renovations, the largest of which were conducted after the Spanish-American War, during World War II, and most recently between 1999 and 2002. Building 1 had provided 169 years of hospital service before it closed to patient care in 1999.

OBJECTIVE

Planning for the new library at NMCP began in earnest in 1994 as libraries nationwide were first experiencing the impact of the online revolution. The challenge was to strike a balance between the traditional library and library of the future. The planners sought to create a library with state-of-the-art technology that demonstrated the Command's commitment to learning and to which users could look with pride. The new facility would accommodate the collections, staff, and services of the Health Sciences Library and the Crew's Library. The objectives of library design included

- comfortable space for study and research,
- adequate space for a growing print collection,
- intuitively useable arrangement of the collection,
- placement of library staff to maximize customer service,
- comfortable office space for the staff,
- expanded computer facilities,
- convenient areas for library equipment,
- meeting spaces, and
- capitalizing on the architectural detail of the historic hospital.

METHODS

Relocating Library Services was part of a major building project that spanned more than a decade. This project included the construction of a new acute care facility and outpatient facilities, renovation of Buildings 1 and 215, and relocation of the administrative offices into the original Naval Hospital. The Medical and Crew's Libraries were to be located in adjacent spaces. Each area was to be outfitted with new furniture and equipment. Planning for the Command-wide construction project managed by the Naval Facilities Engineering Command and the HFPPO of the Naval Healthcare Support Office began in the mid-1980s.

The professional library, then known as the Medical Library, had outgrown its existing space of 3,500 square feet in Building 215. The collection was divided between a main library and a storage area nearby. Crowding had forced the library to drastically weed its collection annually to make room for new materials. Seating space was limited to two easy chairs, five computer workstations, twelve study carrels, and one reading table. Staff space was minimal. The Medical Library's main objective for the new library was to secure adequate space for its collection, staff, and services in a central location within the main hospital.

During the initial phase of space planning, several locations for the libraries were considered. The head medical librarian proposed locating the Medical Library in a centrally located, larger space in the acute care facility. The library space planning guidelines outlined in MLA CE–22, *Planning Hospital Library Facilities,* were used to justify the need for expanded space.[3] The Medical Library's proposal for a location in the main hospital was rejected since the acute care facility was reserved for patient care. By 1992, the Medical Library was assigned a spacious 9,000 square feet in Building 215, although this area spanned two floors and included an internal stairwell.

Two years later, the HFPPO began planning the transformation of Building 1 from a hospital to an administration building. HFPPO proposed placing the Medical Library and Crew's Library in Building 1. Although the Crew's Library had closed, it was included in the renovation plan. The Building 1 location would create libraries with architectural character and state-of-the art technology. The libraries were to be located in a 14,500 square-foot space that included the entire front of the fourth floor along with a perpendicular wing. They were to be adjacent, but separate, each with its own entrance and circulation desks. The Medical Library's 12,000 square-foot space on one floor was remote from the patient care areas.

Fireplaces, archways, original windows with deep windowsills, and wainscoting would add ambience to the libraries. The architects also used Doric columns, mirroring the building portico, to conceal structural beams in the center of the library. Despite the beauty of these architectural assets, the design of the library was constrained by the structure of the building. In the 1830s, buildings relied on their vertical walls for structural integrity. Because the walls and doorways were immovable, planning the interior spaces in Building 1 required fitting function into form.

In December 1995, the library staff reviewed the first set of architectural drawings with the HFPPO team and the architects. By that time the libraries were now slated to operate as one department. It became necessary to move or remove circulation areas, partitions, and entrances. The librarians requested permission to redesign the space. The challenge was to fit the functions of a library accustomed to a small space into a larger, but fragmented space. The library staff tried to take advantage of the partitions imposed by the structure of the building rather than allowing the walls to be stumbling blocks to a workable design.

Although they looked forward to the expanded library spaces, stretching a small staff over a large space required careful planning. The main entrance was placed on the side nearest to the CHCC and the circulation desk was placed close to the main entrance. The reference area was located in the center of the library. Nearby computers make reference assistance readily available to patrons. The reference and circulation areas were positioned to allow direct line of sight between desks so the staff at one desk could easily assist the other. Stack areas, where little assistance is necessary, were placed at ends of the library (see Photo 6.2).

Office space was a priority for the new facility, since the existing Medical Library provided offices for only half of the staff. The fixed sizes of the rooms in Building 1 made it difficult to conform to the Department of Defense facilities planning guidelines that define the size of staff offices. The smaller rooms in the library were not the perfect size to accommodate staff offices. Offices were created in large spaces where new walls could be constructed or in rooms where the spaces could be partitioned. Common staff workspaces, a conference room, and a storage area were incorporated into the design.

In anticipation of the emerging role of technology, the library was equipped with many network connections. Public-access computers were distributed throughout the library, with the largest cluster con-

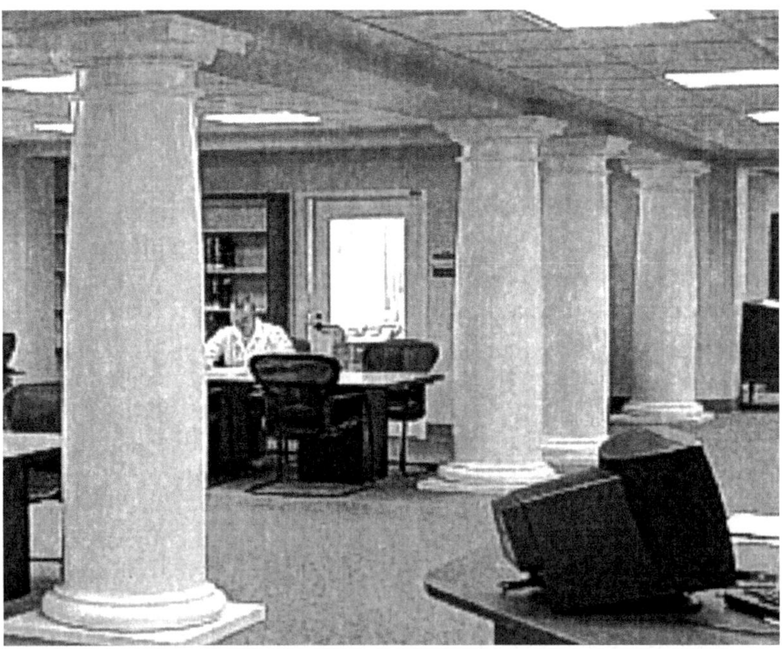

PHOTO 6.2. Library Services reference area. Official U.S. Navy photo.

taining four computers. This arrangement provides the option of private or communal study. To accommodate the need for 24/7 access for the clinical staff, a swipecard security system was installed at the main entrance.

To plan the new shelving, the Medical Library measured its overcrowded shelves of books and journals and calculated the space needed for five years' growth. The floors of the stack areas were reinforced to accommodate conventional library shelving loaded with bound journals, but no provision was made to reinforce the floors for compact shelving. Estimates of the needs of the Crew's Library were made with the assistance of the General Library at Naval Medical Center San Diego. Placement of the shelving accounted for the windows and Americans with Disabilities Act (ADA) guidelines.

In 1996, library staff met with the interior designer to develop a plan for the placement of the furniture, computers, and shelving. The library staff submitted shelving specifications and vendor catalogs to assist the designer in the development of a plan. They worked with the designer to plan the number and placement of the reading tables, study carrels, workstations, computer tables, and easy chairs. Color schemes and artwork for the entire building were selected by HFPPO working with the interior designer. Cherry finish was chosen for the furniture. Library staff selected the upholstery fabric and neutral accent colors in order to achieve a classic look. The interior planning was finished three years before the renovation of Building 1 began and five years before the tentative completion date was in sight (see Figure 6.1).

As the occupancy date for Building 1 drew near, library staff and HFPPO reviewed the shelving plan. In the five years since the finalizing of the original plan the library had expanded to fill the growth room planned earlier. The designer's shelving arrangement was aesthetically pleasing, but inadequate. With HFPPO's permission, library staff consulted a shelving contractor to seek advice on shelving type and placement. Library staff worked with the contractor to reconfigure and add shelving, within budget limits. The library selected interchangeable units for the entire library providing maximum capacity and flexibility of design.

Working from plans with the architects, designer, and shelving contractor was very productive, but nothing replaced the value of walking through the space and matching the plans with reality. Eigh-

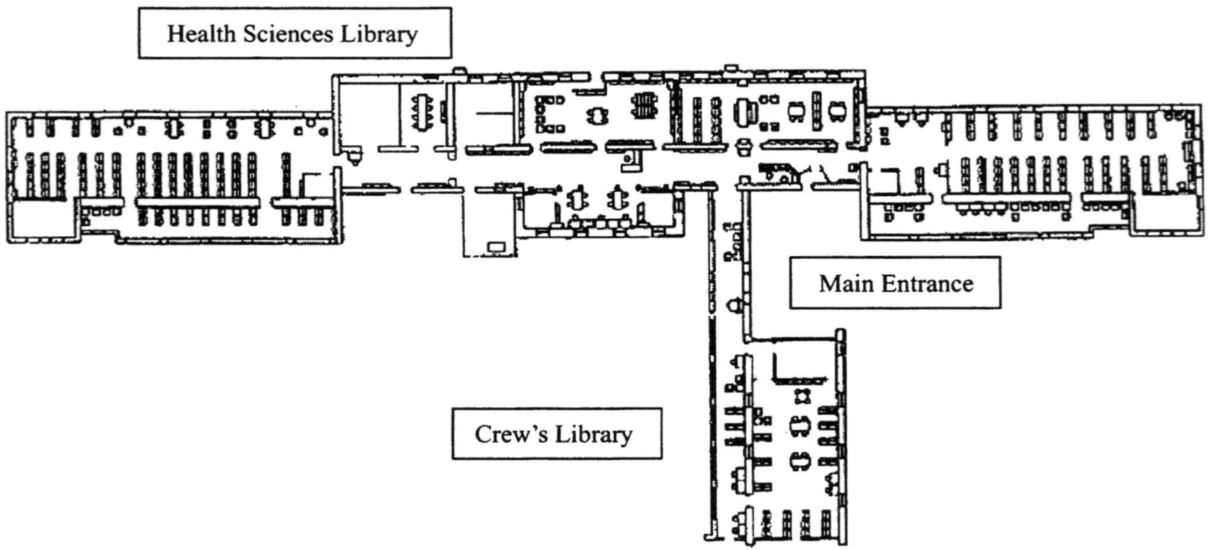

FIGURE 6.1. Building 1 library floor plan. Official U.S. Navy illustration.

teen months prior to occupancy, library staff visited the new spaces for the first time. Although the fourth floor of Building 1 was still a hard hat area, the library was beginning to take shape. During that visit, the staff discovered that the building contractor had decided to expose a fireplace at the end of the stack area in the East Wing. As planned, the shelves would obscure the fireplace. Having selected interchangeable shelving, library staff was able to switch furniture with shelving between two rooms in order to retain shelf space and create a seating area in front of the newly found fireplace.

Six months later, library staff once again visited the library in Building 1. Drywall and carpeting gave the spaces a finished look. As they walked into the stack area on the West Wing, the beauty of the view of the river from the windows was striking. The views of the parking lots from the adjacent Reading Room made it obvious that another reconfiguration of the shelves was necessary. The reading area and stacks were moved to give patrons a marvelous view of the Elizabeth River.

Library staff developed a general collection for the new library. The Command provided some initial funding and reestablished an affiliation with the Navy General Library Program (NGLP). The NGLP facilitated the library's acquisition of a collection from a Navy library that was closing and provided funds to purchase new materials. With the help of volunteers, Library Services staff selected, acquired, cataloged, and processed a core collection for the new Crew's Library.

Four months prior to the move, library staff met with representatives of the moving company to begin planning the move. The major challenges ahead were merging the two journal collections from the main library and storage areas, and the ratio of library staff to moving company staff during the move itself. A detailed map for the placement of the collection in Building 1 was needed to address both challenges. With the help of limited duty military personnel, library staff measured the existing collection in the main library and the archives and estimated the space necessary for five years' growth in the journal collection. Library staff created a map (see Figure 6.2) for the interfiled collection in Building 1 that illustrated the arrangement of the installed shelves in the library stacks. Using the map as a guide, colored signs were placed on each shelf in the new library to aid the library staff and the movers on the proper location of each title. Approximately 2,500 signs were hung in the weeks leading up to the

Move Plan, Shelving

Shelving Range #1 **East Wing**		
AACN Clinical Issues 4 library / 20 growth	Academic Medicine 19 library / 5 growth	Acta Anaes Scan | Acta Cytologica 2 grow | 21 archives / 1 lib
AANA Journal 12 archives / 8 library / 4 growth	Academic Medicine | Academic Psychiatry 10 growth | 5 archives / 5 library/ 4 grow	Acta Cytologica 14 library / 10 growth
AANA Journal | Abdominal Imaging | Academic Emergency Medicine 2 grow | 2 arch / 3 lib | 2 arch / 13 lib / 2 gr	Aca Psy | Acta Anaesthesiologica Scandinavica 1 gro | 23 archives	Acta Endocrinologica 24 archives
Academic Emergency Medicine | Academic Medicine 9 growth | 13 archives / 2 library	Acta Anaesthesiologica Scandinavica 7 archives / 17 library	Acta Endocrinologica 24 archives
EMPTY	Acta Anaesthesiologica Scandinavica 8 library / 16 growth	EMPTY

FIGURE 6.2. Planning map for bound journal placement. Official U.S. Navy illustration.

move. Five library staff members worked with several moving teams of ten each to move the entire collection in seven working days. The intense planning paid off, allowing the library to reopen two days early. When the library opened its doors to users immediately following the completion of the move, it was in perfect order.

RESULTS

The library's greatly anticipated move to expanded spaces on the fourth floor of Building 1 took place in August 2002. The newly renovated facilities tripled the size of the library, allowing a broadening of services to include a Crew's Library and Patient and Family Resource Center. Residents and staff returning from duty assignments elsewhere are amazed at the transformation. The new library offers excellent study areas, a conference room, adequate shelving for the Health Sciences Library books and journals, thirteen public-access computers, and the same familiar faces from Building 215. An electronic swipe-card system offers the staff 24/7 access to the library.

Perception is not everything, but it is very important. The beauty of the renovated spaces changes the way people perceive the library and its services. The number of computers and the arrangement of the collection are in sharp contrast to the old facility. The new spaces make the Health Sciences Library collection and services seem improved. The current journal room displays all subscriptions, allowing hospital staff to find the latest issue of their favorite journals easily and to visually recognize the extent of the current subscriptions. The reorganized and spaciously arranged collection makes the bound journal collection easily accessible. The consolidation of the reference books from the health sciences and general collections brings a wide variety of resources together for easy browsing.

The return of Crew's Library was welcomed by regular library users and brought many new faces to the library. A steady group of regular patrons and new users arrive daily. Many are delighted to find out that the library is not "only for the doctors." Many NMCP staff members are so pleased with the atmosphere and the service in the library that they bring their co-workers on tours and have them register as borrowers.

Patrons come to the library to study, meet, or use the thirteen public-access computers. It is not unusual for all of the stations to be busy. The hospital staff frequently comment on how comfortable it is to come to the library and work without interruption. Visitors tour the building to marvel at its transformation and to reminisce about the past.

CONCLUSION

The wonderful facility enjoyed by many today is the result of a productive collaboration among HFPPO staff, architects, interior designers, and library staff. The HFPPO staff was committed to restoring Building 1 to its dignity as a national historic landmark. The building was stripped to its original walls and carefully rebuilt, creating administrative offices and a library that are the pride of the Command.[4] From blueprints to completion, the library worked closely with HFPPO staff. The librarians contributed their subject expertise and the HFPPO staff brought their reverence for the building and project-management experience. Through careful planning, research, attention to detail, and open dialogue, HFPPO and library staff created a facility better than either could have designed alone. Library staff worked tirelessly to be sure that nothing went unnoticed. Close attention to detail and ongoing modifications within budget guidelines were essential to the success of the renovation.

Frieda Weise, exploring "Library As Place," points out that libraries, beyond being storehouses, are service organizations that embody the mission and vision of their institutions.[5] The new library at NMCP clearly demonstrates the Command's commitment to its vision to be "the center of healthcare excellence in graduate medical education, research and professional growth."[6] Although technology is rapidly changing how information is delivered, it remains important to design libraries that create learning environments that meet users' needs. In reporting the results of the Delphi Study, Ludwig and Starr quote William J. Mitchell, Dean of Architecture and Planning at MIT.[7] Mitchell states that successful spaces focus on light, comfortable surroundings, and views of the outside.[8] The Library Services Department at NMCP is such a space. The commodious atmosphere and state-of-the-art equipment draw patrons to the library. Although it is said that form should follow function, library functions can be comfortably fit into existing space with imagination and an eye for design.

NOTES

1. *The Serendipitous History of Discovery and Development Surrounding the "Hospital Point" Area and Its Naval Hospital in Portsmouth (1558-2000).* Naval Medical Center, Portsmouth, VA. Available online at <http://www-nmcp.mar.med.navy.mil/nmcphist/nmcphist.asp>.

2. Holcomb, Richmond C. *A Century with Norfolk Naval Hospital 1830-1930.* Portsmouth, VA: Printcraft Publishing, 1930: 408.

3. *Planning Hospital Library Facilities,* CE–22. Syllabus. Chicago, IL: Medical Library Association, 1975.

4. Gay, Dan C. "Navy's 'First and Finest' Hospital Rededicated." *Navy Medicine* 94(January-February 2003): 19-20.

5. Weise, Frieda. "Being There: The Library As Place." *Journal of the Medical Library Association* 92(January 2004): 6-13.

6. *Strategic Plan, Naval Medical Center Portsmouth,* January 2004. Available online at <http://www-nmcp.med.navy.mil/StrategicPlan2004.doc>.

7. Ludwig, Logan and Starr, Susan. "Results of a Delphi Study: What the Library Is Depends on What It Does." Presentation at The Library As Place: Symposium on Building and Revitalizing Health Sciences Libraries in the Digital Age, November 5-6, 2003. Available online at <http://www.nlm.nih.gov/building/agenda.html>.

8. "Designing the Space: A Conversation with William J. Mitchell." *Syllabus Magazine* 1(September 2003): 7. Available online at <http://www.syllabus.com/article.asp?id=8105>.

Case Study 7

The Hope Fox Eccles Clinical Library Renovation Project

T. Elizabeth Workman

OVERVIEW

Setting: The Hope Fox Eccles Clinical Library is located at University Hospital (Salt Lake City) and is a branch of the Spencer S. Eccles Health Sciences Library on the University of Utah campus. Opened in 1983, the Clinical Library occupies approximately 1,030 square feet of space. Although the facility was originally designed to exclusively serve clinicians and students, an increasing amount of patrons came to the library seeking consumer health-oriented information. Library staff decided to formally expand the library's mission and strategic plan to address consumer health needs. Library and hospital administration noted the need to update the physical facility.

Objectives: The objectives for the library renovation included creating a more comfortable environment for both consumers and clinicians; improving workspace for staff; maximizing use of space; providing better accommodations for equipment; and improving the overall aesthetics of the facility.

Methods: A university design specialist assessed the library and created several prototype designs. The designer met with the clinical librarian and library director to perfect a particular prototype. Hospital facility and engineering staff began implementation of the design in January 2003. The work of remodeling was completed in two phases, allowing the library to remain open throughout the process. The renovation was completed in March 2003.

Results: The renovation fulfilled all of the project's goals and created a more functional library. A friendly reception area allows staff to greet patrons as they enter. A comfortable conference area creates a place to read and talk. The computer area is more accessible for wheelchairs and intravenous stands. The new carpet, wall covering, and furniture are attractive, comfortable, and inviting.

Conclusions: The Hope Fox Eccles Clinical Library renovation project created a facility that better serves all patrons. Staff members are pleased with the improvements. Overall, the project maximized a relatively small space to function well for several different uses.

INTRODUCTION

Hospital libraries have been a part of the health care scene in the United States since 1763.[1] Today there are thousands of hospital libraries in America. These libraries play a vital role within their institutions. A recent review of several studies indicated that library information had a significant impact on the clinical practice of the physicians surveyed.[2] In the Rochester Study, published in 1992, 94.1 percent of physicians surveyed felt that library services contributed to higher quality care; 19 percent of them went as far as saying library services prevented patient mortality.[3]

Britain G. Roth documented the important role of hospital libraries and health information access in the lives of patients in 1978.[4] Since then, others have published studies on this topic. Several hospital libraries have expanded their mission and goals to formally address the needs of patients and visitors, as well as health professionals. Some libraries fulfill their expanded service missions by creating separate libraries for clinicians and patients, and others combine services to both groups within the same facility.

The Hope Fox Eccles Health Sciences Library, a branch of the Spencer S. Eccles Health Sciences Library, is located within University Hospital on the University of Utah campus in Salt Lake City. The library is staffed from 6:00 a.m. to midnight 365 days a year. Hospital clinicians have 24/7 access to the library.

In May 2002, in response to increasing needs for patient and consumer-oriented health information, the Clinical Library formally expanded its mission and strategic plan to provide optimal service to all of its patrons. Recognizing the need to remodel the facility to better serve patrons, library staff identified specific goals and outcomes for the renovation project. The following year, workers completely renovated the library to accommodate a variety of patron groups.

Historic Background

The need for clinical literature has always extended beyond the walls of traditional academic libraries. In 1942, when the Salt Lake County General Hospital agreed to accommodate the clinical learning needs of University of Utah medical students, an ad hoc collection soon formed on-site to serve in place of medical texts located several miles away in the central library on campus. When University Hospital was built on the University of Utah campus in 1965, a portion of the adjacent College of Medicine wing became a separate, independent library and the health sciences collection was relocated from central campus. This space served its purpose until the completion of the Spencer S. Eccles Health Sciences Library, a new facility located just yards from the Hospital/College of Medicine structure. In 1981, the construction of a new hospital north of the original facility recreated a sizable distance between students, clinical staff, and the library. A satellite library opened within the new University Hospital in April 1983 to reconcile the distance issue. From the beginning, the Hope Fox Eccles Clinical Library has not only served patrons with its print collection, on-site staff, and computers, but also acted as a conduit to the more extensive resources at the main health sciences library. Patrons have access to these resources via messenger or telephone.

Although the facility was originally designed to serve clinicians and students exclusively, the library never turned away patients seeking health information. Before the availability of consumer health information, library staff had to rely on professional literature to serve most patient information needs. With the popular advent of more consumer-friendly health information, staff members better served patients with materials that were easier to read. However, in the first years of operation, library clientele mainly consisted of hospital health care providers and students.

In recent years, with increasing numbers of patients seeking consumer health-oriented information, library staff decided to formally expand the library's mission and strategic plan to address consumer health needs. The Clinical Library composed the following mission statement:

> Our mission is to provide quality health information services to the patients, visitors, and staff of University Hospital and the general community. We gladly assist patients, their families, and other visitors in finding the information they need, in addition to providing library services to hospital staff.

Library staff adopted the following set of general service provisions:

- Assist university staff and students in finding information needed for patient care, education, and research.
- Provide information services for patients and their families, plus visitors from the general community.
- Provide a facility where people may access the Internet.
- Provide trained staff to assist all patrons in finding information.
- Partner with other hospital groups to provide information services to everyone, at the point of need.

Library staff drafted a new plan to document and utilize specific strategies to serve patrons seeking consumer health information, with expected outcomes. Strategies and outcomes included:

Strategy: Market patient information services by supplying handouts to all waiting areas and clinics.

Outcome: More patients and other laypersons will visit the library; patients will have a tangible item that communicates services, facility highlights, and hours of operation.

Strategy: Meet with hospital staff to inform them about services.

Outcome: Informed hospital staff will encourage patients to visit the library; hospital staff patronage will also increase.

Strategy: Strategize with hospital administration to identify "target areas" (clinics, units, waiting areas) where patients and visitors will find library services especially appealing.
Outcome: Increased patronage, and better-informed patients and visitors.

Strategy: Partner with other service groups (i.e., rehabilitation) to serve their patients' specific needs.
Outcome: Specialized services for individual patient groups.

To gauge the success of the planned service expansion, library staff also monitored other statistics such as types and instances of reference requests, computer use, and ratio of layperson and health professional patronage. Library and hospital administration also noted the need to update the physical facility to adequately serve all patron groups, and to bring the facility into the new millennium.

FACILITY RENOVATION—PHYSICAL DESCRIPTION

The Clinical Library includes approximately 1,030 square feet of space and has occupied the same area since it opened in 1983. Before the renovation, the library had retained much of the same look and feel from its original design. The total space was divided into two general areas. A large area housed three rows of stacks and most of the study carrels. The smaller half largely functioned as a staff workspace. In this design, the stacks area served as a built-in barrier that protected study carrels from conversations and the noise of the copier. The design also provided adequate workspace for staff, although it slightly isolated them from patrons. A large conference table with shelving for indices bridged the two areas and provided ample surface space for working with a predominantly print collection (see Figure 7.1).

Renovation Objectives

Library staff and administration noted specific goals and desired outcomes including the following:

- *More comfortable environment for both consumer and clinician patron groups.* Library staff recognized that patients and health professionals have different needs. Although clinicians felt more comfortable in the library's research environment, patients and other visitors needed a "less clinical" setting to ease what is usually an emotionally heightened period in their lives. Patrons dealing with an acute health crisis needed a warmer, more "homelike" setting.
- *Improved workspace for staff.* Staff recognized the opportunity to improve workspaces in the forms of counter surfaces, storage space, and work area placement. The new design would optimally integrate the staff work area with patron space to better facilitate service. Cabinet space could be upgraded. Increased surface area would also better accommodate equipment, such as scanners, in addition to giving staff more space to complete various tasks.
- *Maximized use of space.* Since the Clinical Library is housed in a relatively small area, staff welcomed the opportunity to improve the use of the entire space. The design team studied the stacks, computer area, study places, and staff areas to harmonize the way in which these individual spaces worked together, and to optimize the functionality of the entire library.
- *Better accommodations for equipment.* Although the library did not house many computers or other equipment, the existing hardware needed to be regrouped to complement the different functions of the library. Factors to consider included: who used the equipment and the needs of these individuals, noise generated by equipment, and otherwise how it affected patrons, staff, and their needs in both negative and positive ways.
- *Overall aesthetic improvement of the facility.* The design team sought to use the existing strengths of the facility while updating its look. The angular shape of the room had potential for appearing more open. The large window overlooking the Salt Lake Valley could be made more accessible to everyone. Carpet, wall coverings, and other furnishings needed to be updated to create an inviting library to serve diverse patron groups. The library needed more chairs and casual meeting space for patients and their visitors.

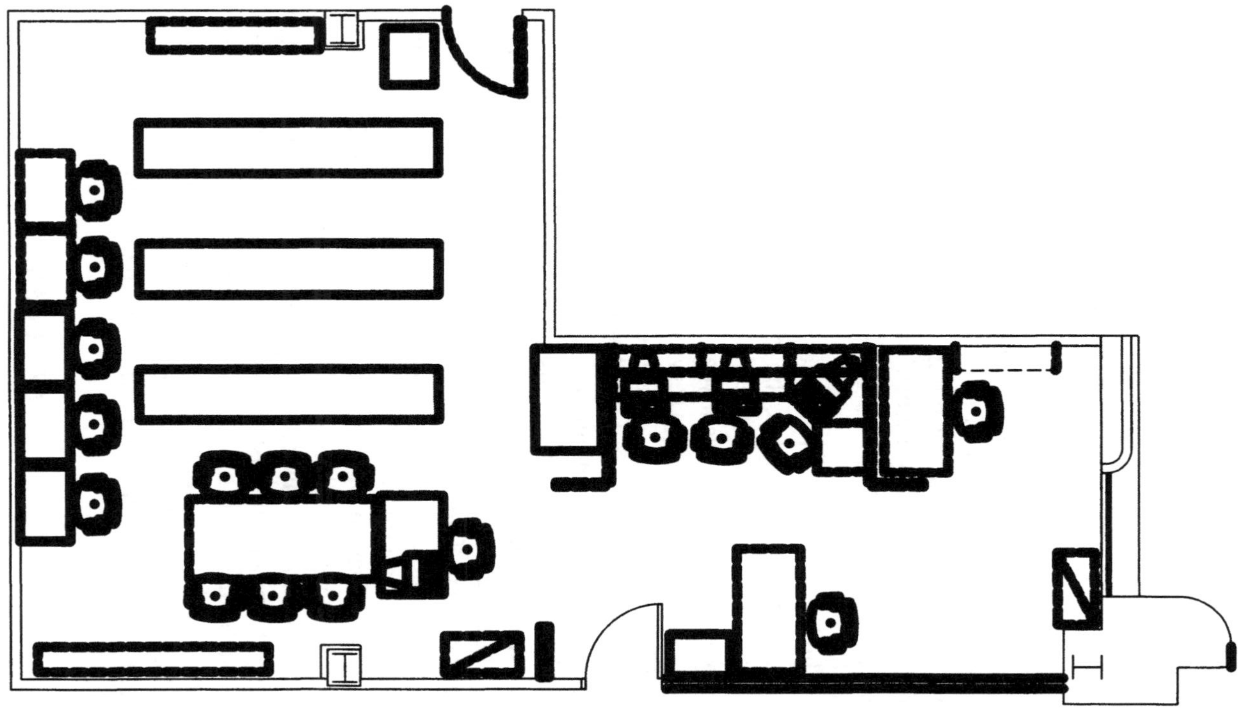

FIGURE 7.1. Library layout prior to renovation. Drawn by Kathy Sirrine. Reprinted with permission.

METHODS

A university design specialist assessed the library and created several prototype designs. The designer, clinical librarian, and library director held multiple meetings to perfect a particular prototype. This prototype fulfilled all of the goals and suggested additional spatial and functional improvements. The design team implemented creative and practical strategies to fulfill the specific goals within the same limited space.

The Eccles family and the hospital's Volunteer Auxiliary provided all the funding to complete the renovation. Hospital facility and engineering staff began implementing the design in January 2003. The library is staffed 365 days a year, from 6:00 a.m. to midnight, to provide essential information services, and is accessible to hospital staff 24/7 for research needs. To avoid service interruption, workers completed the renovation in two phases, and the library retained its normal schedule throughout the process. This was accomplished by dividing the library into two areas with a temporary barrier. Construction workers entered each area and transported tools and materials through a separate door. This minimized noise and disturbance on library patrons. Throughout the process, the only time the library closed during business hours was when the new carpet was laid and its adhesive dried, and this was accomplished in just a few hours.

The renovation was completed in March 2003. The library held an open house to introduce patrons to the new facility. This event coincided with the official public open house of the new emergency care wing at University Hospital, creating an opportunity for library staff to reach out to the many visitors who were in the hospital for this event. During the library open house, staff introduced many visitors and clinicians alike to the library's services, and communicated to them how the library could improve their overall health experience.

OUTCOMES

The renovation addressed all of the design team's original goals. Many strategies to improve overall comfort were implemented. The designer assembled a newer, warmer, more inviting color scheme for the carpet, wall covering, and furniture. The blinds on the large window overlooking the Salt Lake Valley were removed to increase natural light, which made this window an inviting, comfortable place for reading and conversing. A reception desk and counter were placed directly across from the entrance, enabling staff to greet patrons as they entered the library. Before the renovation, library staff did not enjoy immediate eye contact with patrons. The reception counter area also provided improved space for staff computers, printers, plus shelf space for essential work documentation.

Workers removed the conference table and installed two smaller, less formal circular tables for the window and stacks area. This created more open space and a more homelike appearance for patients. All staff furniture was replaced with new, more workable modular desk space. The modular furniture provided more under-the-counter space for filing cabinets, computer towers, surge protectors, and other essential items.

The clinical librarian's desk was replaced with modular furniture that supplied more surface and storage space. The relocation also placed the librarian closer to patrons, to better serve them. Workers removed old storage facilities and replaced them with customized floor-to-ceiling cabinets that provided more space and were less obtrusive. Flip-style cabinets were installed above work areas and the patrons' computer area provided ample storage space for paper and other supplies. The computer area was slightly reconfigured, with the stand-alone workstation placed in an area more convenient for wheelchair patrons.

Blinds were removed from the floor-to-ceiling windows between the library and hospital hallway. This provided more visual access to the computer area from the hallway. Passersby noted the computers and inquired about the library's services.

The library inhabited a relatively small area, so the design team made some changes to maximize the use of all space. The first of the three stacks was reduced from a full-sized stack to a half-height shelving unit. The top of this midsized stack provided much of the surface area formerly provided by the large table. This change also created a more open feeling.

Workers moved the wall display for new journal issues near the librarian's new work area, for improved access and visual effect. The photocopier was moved near the entrance, which made it more accessible to patrons and staff yet distancing it from quiet study areas. All computer towers were moved under counters, which provided more protection from spills and other accidents. The printer was moved to a better location behind the reception counter. The electrician moved the patron telephone closer to the entrance, for better access.

The new carpet, wall coverings, furniture, and new configurations greatly improved the library's ambience. New art prints and an original work from a local artist adorned the walls (see Figure 7.2).

Statistical Outcomes

Staff monitored statistical markers to measure success. These included types and instances of reference requests, computer use, and ratio of layperson and health professional patronage.

Reference Requests

Overall reference work has increased. In comparing January 2004 requests to those of January 2003, there was a 215 percent increase in reference requests. There has also been a significant increase in requests from patients and visitors.

Computer Use

Since the renovation, computer use has increased 133 percent. Once the library expanded its service mission, computer use began to dramatically climb. Staff also noted changing trends in types of computer use. E-mail use quickly increased, as did research for consumer-oriented information.

Patronage

A two-week sample study conducted in February 2004 illustrated that both patron groups use the library in an almost even ratio. Approximately 47.5 percent of patrons were patients or visitors, and 52.5 percent were clinicians or other university affiliates. Although a study of this kind had not been done prior to the renovation, staff have observed a greater balance between the layperson and health professional groups. The facility improvements also attracted new clinicians to the library.

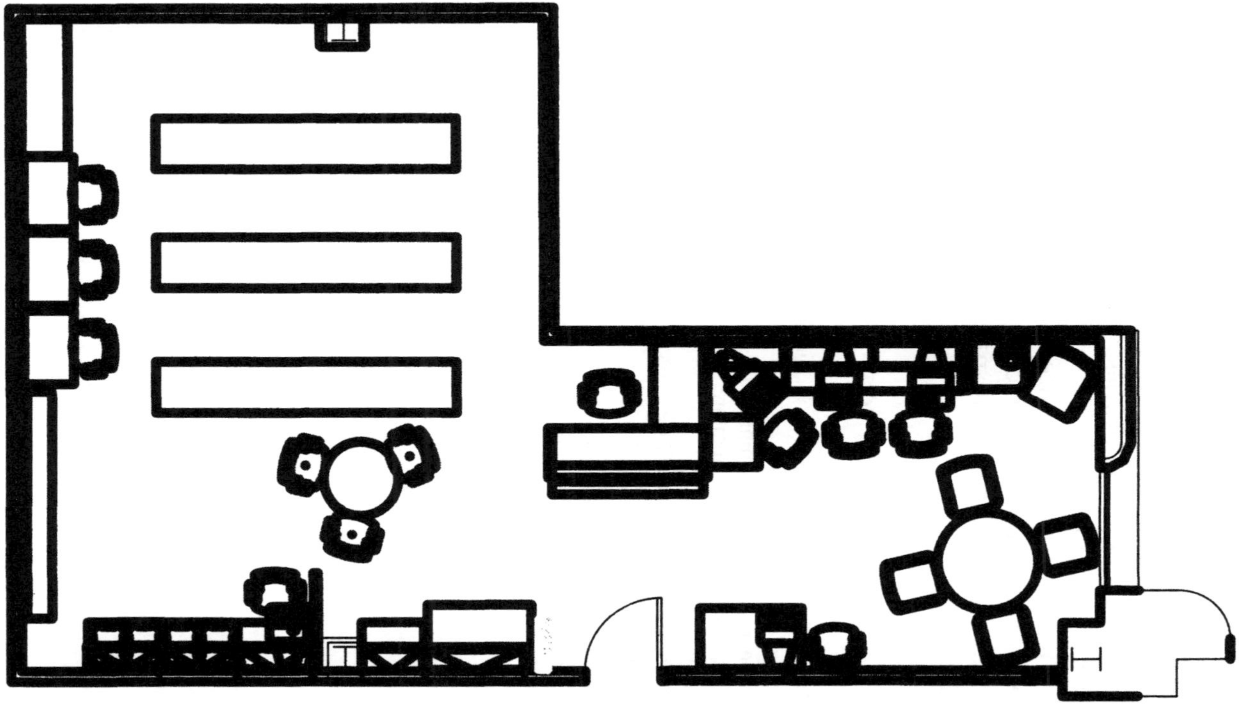

FIGURE 7.2. Library layout after renovation was completed. Drawn by Kathy Sirrine. Reprinted with permission.

CONCLUSION

The Hope Fox Eccles Clinical Library renovation project created a facility that better serves all patrons. Quantitative indicators and observation show that the renovation has helped achieve the anticipated outcomes for the expanded service mission and its strategic goals. Staff members are pleased with the improvements. Overall, the project maximized a relatively small space to function well for several different uses.

NOTES

1. Holst, Ruth. "Hospital Libraries in Perspective." *Bulletin of the Medical Library Association* 79(January 1991):1-9.

2. O'Connor, Patrick. "Determining the Impact of Health Library Services on Patient Care: A Review of the Literature." *Health Information and Libraries Journal* 19(March 2002):1-13.

3. Marshall, Joanne G. "The Impact of the Hospital Library on Clinical Decision Making: The Rochester Study." *Bulletin of the Medical Library Association* 80 (April 1992):169-178.

4. Roth, Britain G. "Health Information for Patients: The Hospital Library's Role." *Bulletin of the Medical Library Association* 66(January 1978):14-18.

PART III: ACADEMIC MEDICAL CENTER LIBRARIES

Case Study 8

Managing a Library Renovation Project: A Team Approach

Deanna M. Lucia
Mary E. Piorun

OVERVIEW

Setting/resources: The Lamar Soutter Library is a midsized academic health science library. The library employs forty-one full-time employees and occupies 41,000 square feet within the University of Massachusetts Medical School. The library renovation budget was $1.5 million.

Objective: The goal of the library renovation was to improve the functionality of user service points, increase overall comfort, improve the general appearance, and update staff and public areas to incorporate current advances in technology. The library has used a team-based approach to operational problem solving since 1998. Use of this team structure allowed the inclusion of faculty, students, administration, and library staff in the renovation project.

Methods: In 1998, the first Facilities Team was formed to look at the condition of the library and recommend both short- and long-term improvements. Four other teams were created and given charges ranging from studying building options to following up with problems after the renovation was completed. Teams included representatives from all library departments and from a variety of university departments.

Results: Completed in spring 2003, the renovation project successfully improved the library's physical space by offering more seating options, better lighting, and increased accessibility to the library's resources. Staff work areas were also enhanced by organizing staff by department and creating an open work environment that is more conducive to collaboration.

Conclusion: The team-based approach included faculty, staff, and students in the decision-making process throughout the project, and gave them a sense of ownership and pride for the "new" library. Team-based decisions created staff buy-in and staff support of renovation changes. Involving staff and users proved to be invaluable in completing a project that truly met the needs of the library's users.

INTRODUCTION

In 1998, the Lamar Soutter Library of the University of Massachusetts Medical School introduced a team-based approach to problem solving. Pilot teams were formed on a variety of topics ranging from staff development to outreach and education. The first facilities team was formed as a part of this pilot project. Because this team was a success, it became the foundation for four future remodel teams: the space study team, remodel planning team, remodel implementation team, and remodel follow-up team.

Library management believed that having staff members and library users involved with all future facilities teams would help create buy-in to facilities projects, and would allow all changes to focus on the needs of the people using the library's services and staff work spaces. Expanding team membership to include staff members from across library departments, external architects, and staff from other university departments allowed teams to capitalize on a diverse set of skills and lead to more creative problem solving.

Setting/Resources

Founded in 1976, the Lamar Soutter Library is a midsized academic health science library that serves the University of Massachusetts Medical School's School of Medicine, Graduate School of Nursing, and Graduate School of Biomedical Sciences. At the start of the renovation project in 1999, there were thirty-seven full-time equivalent (FTE) employees, and the library housed 625,000 volumes in 41,318 square feet.

Encompassing three floors, the library surrounds a three-story atrium with skylights designed to be the primary source of light in the principal study area. The library is accessed from one entrance on the first floor of the Medical School. The circulation and reference desks are both located near this entrance. The first floor contains the book collection, government documents, and current journals, as well as staff workspaces for reference, access services, systems, and technical services departments. Library administrative offices are located on the second floor, which also offers a mezzanine area for studying and fifty-six individual study carrels for students. An additional fifty-six study carrels are located on the third floor. Bound journals are shelved on the second and third floors.

Prior to the renovation, the circulation desk was constructed of wood, cement, and granite, and the reference desk was made of traditional modular furniture. Seventy-five computer terminals were located in the front section of the library's first floor and were separated by a six-foot wall that obstructed visibility across the floor (see Photos 8.1 and 8.2).

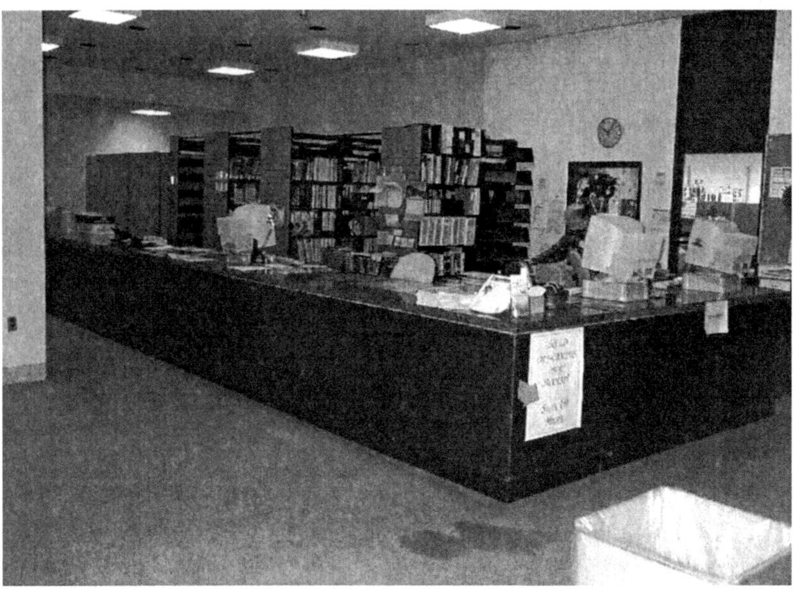

PHOTO 8.1. Prerenovation circulation desk. Photo by Mary E. Piorun. Reprinted with permission.

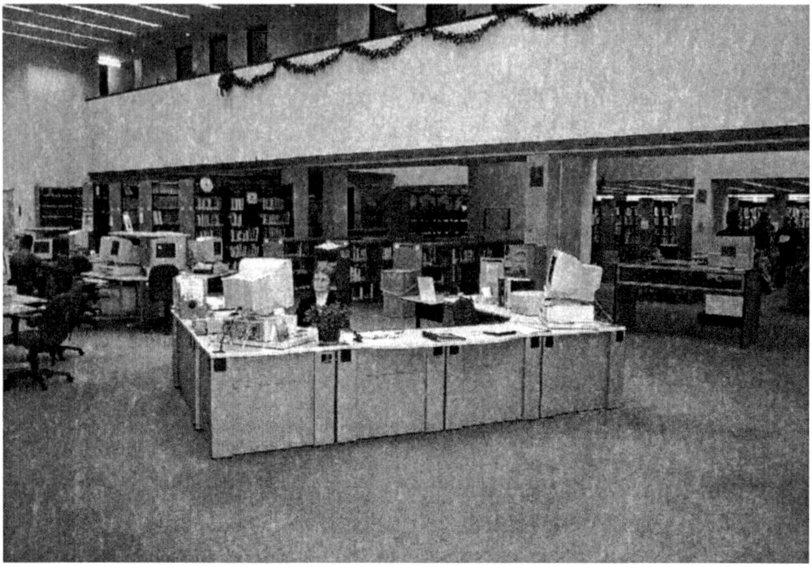

PHOTO 8.2. Prerenovation reference desk. Photo by Mary E. Piorun. Reprinted with permission.

The library's location within the Medical School building adds to its high annual visitor rate of approximately 400,000 students, researchers, clinicians, and members of the public. For students, the library has always been more than a place to study by serving as the only computing center on campus and functioning as the school's social center. This "social center" atmosphere sometimes conflicts with the needs of researchers and clinicians when noise travels from the first floor to the third floor, making it difficult to find quiet space for research and study.

Although the library frequently experimented with relocating collections and service points, and added network cabling whenever possible, an overall plan was not developed to accommodate the growing collection and changes in technology. By the 1990s, the growth of the collection made it increasingly difficult to shelve books and journals. The number of staff members had grown along with the collection, which meant that staff members were forced to share workspaces, and members of the same department were not always seated together because of limited space and poor office layouts. Tall partitions in some areas isolated staff from one another and made it difficult for air to circulate properly.

Objective

The overall objective of the renovation project was to improve the functionality of the library for both staff members and patrons by using a team-based approach to the project's planning, management, and implementation. This approach was important to library management, who believed that consulting with staff and library users about their needs and desires would result in the most effective improvements to the facility.

Consultations with library staff members revealed that in order to perform their jobs more effectively, they needed to work in areas organized by department with their manager's office in close proximity to their workspace. Systems, technical services, and access services staff needed more space. The systems department did not have enough storage space for equipment or the means to secure it properly. In the technical services area, a more open work environment was desired, because workflow (unpacking, sorting, processing, and arranging of materials for cataloging) and collaboration were hindered by the high partitions between workplaces. Access services staff needed room for printers, fax machines, and photocopiers, and secure areas to store laptops and personal items. Because most access services staff shared work areas, additional computer workstations were required to perform off-desk duties. The access services department also needed additional shelving for reserve materials and requested locating the circulation desk closer to the library entrance for better oversight and control of items leaving the library.

Library staff sought to design more effective areas for both formal and informal bibliographic instruction, as well as areas for small group study and collaboration. To meet patrons' computing needs, the library hoped to increase the number of computing stations, upgrade the wireless network, and increase the number of data ports for laptops. The library also recognized a need to create identifiable public service desks placed in locations that would be easy for patrons to find, and that would be located centrally to the materials needed for efficient operations. Additional shelving was needed to accommodate the growing collection and to provide collection layout options that focused on patron needs. Patrons also requested noise reduction between floors. Finally, the renovation sought to provide a more open and welcoming atmosphere with an updated look and more options for comfortable seating and better lighting (see Photos 8.3 and 8.4).

Throughout the renovation process, library staff communicated with patrons regarding current and future facility changes. The status of library services remained a priority. It was imperative to keep the library open throughout the entire renovation and to continuously apprise patrons of changes that affected services or collections.

METHODS

Library management was committed to using a team model in managing the renovation project, and issued a formal charge to each

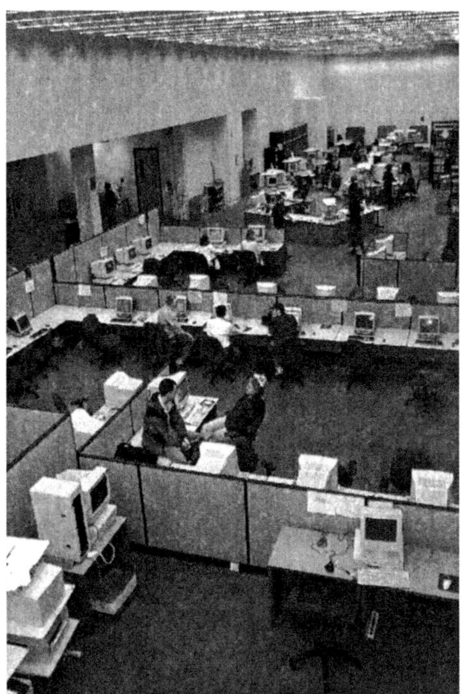

PHOTO 8.3. Prerenovation computing area. Photo by Mary E. Piorun. Reprinted with permission.

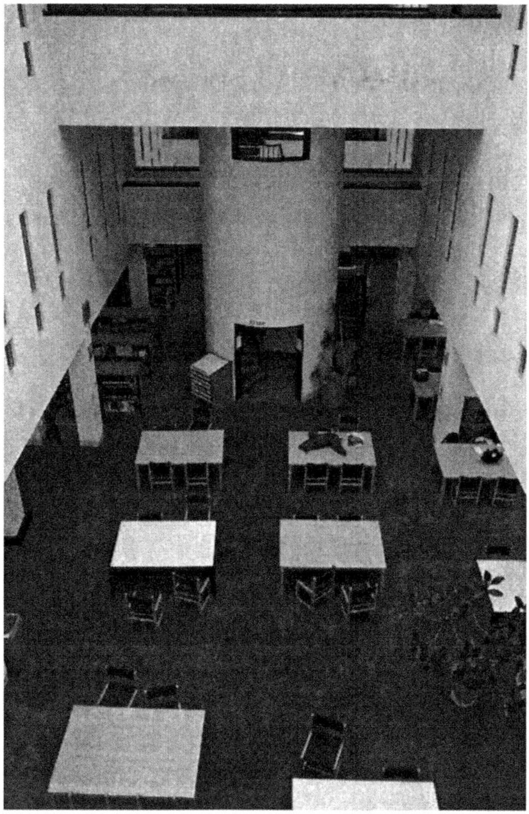

PHOTO 8.4. Prerenovation study tables. Photo by Mary E. Piorun. Reprinted with permission.

team. Each team was assigned a chairperson who called meetings to order and set an agenda for each meeting; a champion who worked with the team chairperson to bring formal requests to management; and team members. Teams consisted of library staff and, when appropriate, people from outside of the library. Library management tried to match individual talents with project needs to assemble the most productive and successful teams possible. Through the formation of five teams, each with its own objective, the library worked through the planning process, developed an implementation timeline, and handled the issues of day-to-day project management.

Facilities Team, 1998-1999

First formed in 1998, the facilities team operated before renovation planning began. This team was charged with considering particular facilities issues that could be addressed immediately within the library's operating budget and recommending ways to resolve each issue. The team also identified renovation changes that would require budgeting and approval from Medical School administration. Facilities team membership was limited to library staff.

Space Study Team, 1999-2000

A space study team was created by school administration in 1999 to address the issues raised by the facilities team. The facilities department assigned an official project manager to work on the library renovation project. This project manager chaired the space study team; team membership consisted primarily of school administration personnel. The charge of the space study team was to propose and evaluate options that would meet the needs of library services and collection requirements, taking into consideration expected growth and future technological advances. Any number of options could be proposed, but the team needed to consider cost, time frame, state construction process requirements, ADA compliance, and to take into account larger campus modernization projects. The team recognized the unique skills needed to meet the charge and determined it would be best to outsource the space study to professional architects. *The Medical Library Study* was conducted over one calendar year. This document presented numerous options for renovation including remodeling the current space, building an addition, and building a new library within a new research building. School administration chose to renovate the existing library. This option was agreed upon with the understanding that within ten years, a new library would be constructed in a newly planned research building on the Medical School campus.

Remodel Planning Team, 2000-2001

In fall 2000, the remodel planning team was formed to design the new layout and aesthetics of the Library as proposed in *The Medical Library Study.* Membership for this team consisted of architects, a facilities project manager, management-level library staff, and various representatives from other school departments, such as telecommunications and networking.

With the formation of the remodel planning team, the library renovation project became a reality. After two years of planning, everyone was excited about being involved in the planning process and looked forward to future changes. The scope of the project was larger than any library team had taken on in the past, but there were clear limits set on this team: one year to propose a design, and a budget of $1.5 million.

The team was responsible for advocating the needs of the library staff and users. Working with the architects, focus groups were conducted with library staff, students, and faculty to learn what people liked about the current library and what improvements needed to be made. The architects examined each task performed by library staff and determined the amount of space necessary to perform that task efficiently. With this knowledge, the architects then experimented with various layouts for office spaces.

The planning team made many purchasing and operational decisions related to furniture, fabrics, color scheme, operating a single reference/circulation desk or two separate desks, building a small group study area and a larger instructional room in existing space, and the overall layout of the entire library. Some of these decisions were based on the input from staff and patrons, and others were made by team members for logistical reasons. The team was often faced with making difficult choices between two desired outcomes, and it became clear that some of the items on the library's "wish list" would have to wait until the new library had been constructed.

Remodel Implementation Team, 2001-2002

To implement the designs created by the remodel planning team, the remodel implementation team was formed in 2001. This team was made up of three permanent members: Director of Library Services; Associate Director of Systems for the Library; and the Facilities Project Manager, and other library managers who attended team meetings when the topic for discussion affected their department. The implementation team also met with representatives from school departments (information services, telecommunications, etc.) and outside vendors when appropriate.

The Facilities Project Manager served as the liaison for the planning team with all contractors and vendors. All changes to plans written by the remodel planning team had to be approved through the Facilities Project Manager, because this person was ultimately responsible for making sure that the project stayed on schedule, was implemented according to plan, and was completed within the approved $1.5 million budget.

The implementation team was responsible for establishing and adjusting a timeline to ensure minimal disruption for students and faculty. This timeline for the overall project was created early in the team's existence and provided a framework for the major construction phases that would be completed throughout the remodel project. At each meeting, the team used this master timeline to formulate detailed project timelines for each specific area of construction to be performed in the following week. The detailed project timelines allowed for the numerous changes in construction schedules, delivery of furniture, etc.

The implementation team was also responsible for keeping library patrons and staff informed of how the construction process would affect them on a daily/weekly basis. To achieve this goal, poster-board signs were placed at the library entrance detailing remodel progress and which library services were affected. These signs also indicated the predicted noise level for the day, giving patrons the option to pick up free earplugs at the circulation desk if they needed some quiet study time. The display case outside of the library entrance provided patrons with information about the remodel project, as did the library's newsletter, the *SoutteReview.* The Director of Library Services provided the library staff with a weekly update regarding the status of the remodel project and what to expect in the near future.

Remodel Follow-Up Team, 2002-2003

After the major aspects of the renovation had been completed, some unresolved issues remained. The remodel follow-up team was created in 2002 to identify problems resulting from the remodel project and to look at building aesthetics and make recommendations regarding signage, artwork, plants, etc. Every department in the library was asked to volunteer one staff member to the follow-up team, so that concerns from each department could be addressed at team meetings.

The follow-up team inspected the library and surveyed other library staff members to find all problem areas such as spaces that had not been painted, carpet and furniture that was either damaged or had been installed incorrectly, furniture that did not match what had been ordered, and defective items. Once problem areas were identified and included on the team's "punch list," the team needed to determine how to best resolve the problems so that the chairperson could take action to correct the problems through the Facilities Project Manager. The remodel project was not considered officially complete until every item on the punch list was corrected.

Because all signage had been removed during the renovation project, the follow-up team created a proposal to replace it, calling for two types: room signage (which had to conform to Medical School standards), and directional signage (which would be created by the architects who designed the remodel plans). Due to budgetary constraints, the proposal has not been implemented yet.

Artwork for the library was not included in the remodel budget, but the follow-up team felt strongly that the large expanses of blank walls needed some artwork to make the atmosphere less "institutional." The library decided to form a relationship with the Medical School's development office, which is in charge of displaying the works of local artists throughout the school. For a minimal cost, the library was able to install hanging strips and hooks, and to serve as another display location within the Medical School.

Although the follow-up team had what many considered the least-exciting charge of the remodel teams, this team's work was invaluable to the overall project. At a time when everyone was ready to consider the project completed (particularly the outside vendors and contractors), the team solved problems that could easily have been overlooked and forgotten but would have led to a less successful and complete renovation.

RESULTS

The renovation project and its follow up were completed in spring 2003, and marked by a rededication celebration in April 2003. The completed renovation project successfully satisfied many of the identified needs voiced by the library's patrons and staff. The entire staff of the access services department, which includes interlibrary loan and circulation functions, is now located behind the circulation desk, near the front entrance. The circulation desk provides staff with locked cabinets for their personal items and locked storage areas for laptops, supplies, etc. The circulation desk provides ample room for fax machines, scanners, and printers. Off-desk workstations have increased from one to three. The systems department acquired approximately 400 square feet of space from an area that was previously occupied by the Graduate School of Nursing. This additional space allowed systems to store computer equipment in a secure location. The small cubicles with high walls in the technical services area were transformed into larger, more open spaces that encourage staff collaboration. Shelving space for technical services was also increased (see Photos 8.5 and 8.6).

In addition to the improvements made in the library's staff spaces, the renovation also enhanced public areas. The general computing area was redesigned to offer users more privacy while working and

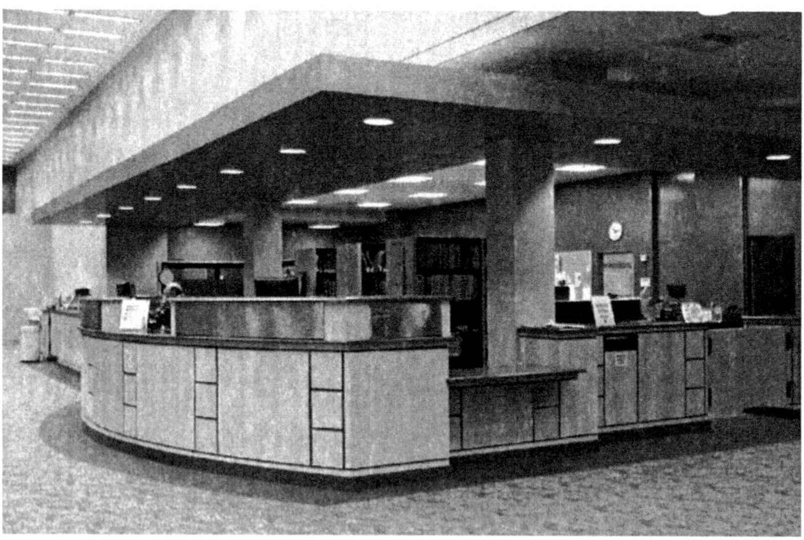

PHOTO 8.5. Postrenovation circulation desk. Photo by Lynn Borella. Reprinted with permission.

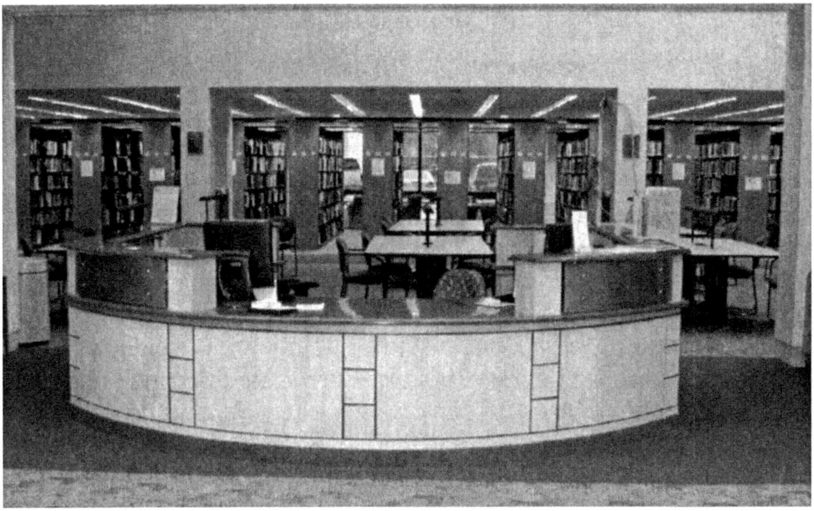

PHOTO 8.6. Postrenovation reference desk. Photo by Lynn Borella. Reprinted with permission.

sufficient workspace while using the computers. Low panels replaced the high partitions between workstations to capitalize on the natural light from the library's atrium. The new circulation and reference desks were both custom-built with common design elements, to be recognized as service points and to better accommodate the needs of both patrons and staff. An audiovisual area was constructed with eight individual viewing stations. Patrons can watch videotapes in a newly constructed group viewing room, which also doubles as a much-needed group study area. Assorted comfortable seating options were placed throughout the library. Improved lighting was added wherever possible, including lighting and electricity at study tables. Soundproof panels were added to the library's walls and walkways over the main atrium to help muffle conversations and keyboard typing. Overall, the color scheme was changed from dated polyester orange and blue to earth tones. The centralized photocopy room was dismantled and photocopiers were relocated throughout the three floors of the library, placing the copiers closer to points of need within the journal stacks. The vacated space of the former photocopy room was transformed into a state-of-the-art computer classroom for library instructional services with seating for twenty students, and a smaller, informal training area was built for small group instruction (see Photos 8.7 and 8.8).

The renovation did not address all of the needs of the library's staff and patrons. Building codes prevented the construction of more group study rooms. Although the circulation desk is adjacent to the library's entrance, staff members still feel that the design of the desk does not allow them to process materials close to the security gate and keep the rest of the library in their line of sight. The purchase of a new gate is currently being considered, as is moving the current gate so that it will be closer to the main service point of the circulation desk. As mentioned earlier, library signage was not included in the renovation budget and has not yet been created. Funds for additional atrium lighting were not included in the renovation budget, but alternate funding allowed installation of additional fixtures to supplement natural light.

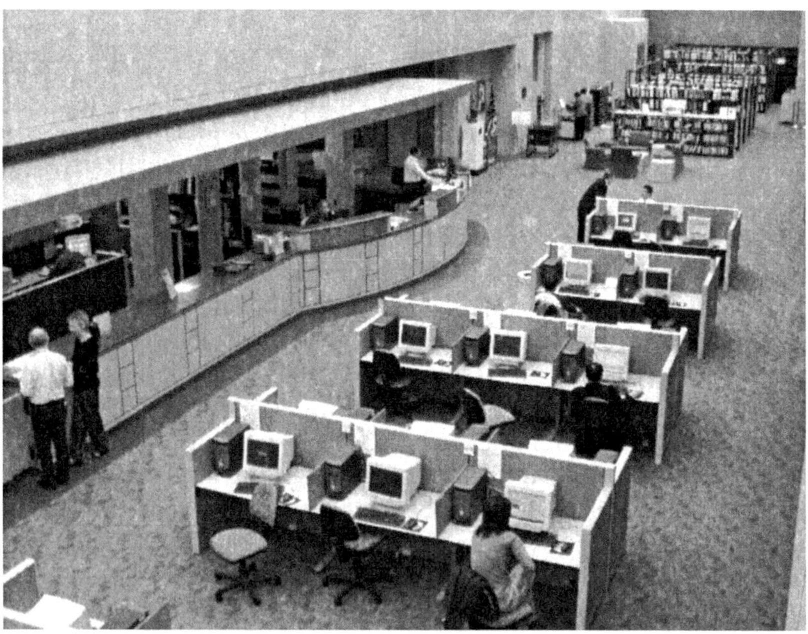

PHOTO 8.7. Postrenovation computing area. Photo by Mary E. Piorun. Reprinted with permission.

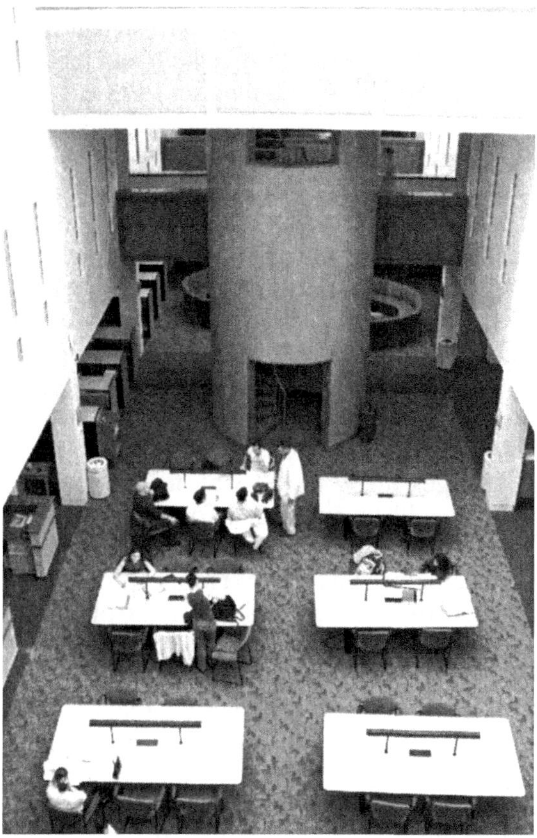

PHOTO 8.8. Postrenovation study tables. Photo by Lynn Borella. Reprinted with permission.

CONCLUSION

Involving many people in the renovation project through the use of teams resulted in a longer project from start to finish, but this increased project length was well worth the benefits that each of the five renovation teams provided. Involving staff members and patrons in the renovation process allowed troubleshooting to occur during the project rather than at its conclusion. Decisions made in the team structure created staff buy-in, so that when it came time to implement renovation changes, staff supported the changes. The team-based approach included faculty, staff, and students in the decision-making process and gave them a sense of ownership and pride for the "new" library. For the first time in the library's twenty-eight years of existence, it was featured on the cover of the Medical School's catalog for the 2003-2005 academic years.

Despite the success of the renovation project, the library's need for space planning has not ended. Because the library did not gain extra square footage for collection storage, a team has been created to address the future space needs of the library's growing book and journal collections. Planning has also begun for the creation of the new library as proposed in *The Medical Library Study.*

Because of the success of the five remodel teams, the construction process for the new library will also be managed using the team approach. Learning from the shortcomings of the remodel teams, there will be some changes made to the way teams operate for the new building project. It will be important for the construction teams to take and save minutes from each meeting. Because meeting minutes were not recorded, many steps of the remodel processes are not documented. Staff will also be more involved on the planning team for the new library. Due to staff vacancies, some departments were not always represented on the remodel planning team, which meant that the implementation team was forced to return to the planning phase when staff felt that the designs for their area were not suitable for their work.

Overall, the same process will be followed, because taking the time to study, plan, implement, and follow up was essential to the success of the project. Involving staff and users also proved to be invaluable in completing a project that truly met the needs of the library's users.

Case Study 9

Continuous Library Facility Improvement at the University of New Mexico Health Sciences Library and Informatics Center

Janis Teal
Holly Shipp Buchanan

OVERVIEW

Setting: In 1997 the Vice President for Health Sciences at the University of New Mexico (UNM) announced an expanded role for and the creation of a new academic and research technology development unit within the library. These programmatic and functional changes required significant changes to the library's form and facilities both to advance technologically and to respond to staff office and collection issues in a 40,000 square-foot space, which was too small for its expanded role.

Objectives: Phase I of the renovation plan was a three-year capital-funded initiative titled Library 2000 Project, which created new spaces for computer use and computer-based instruction, doubled staff size, and improved collection access. Subsequent phases required annual, diversified, internal funding.

The authors wish to thank the staff of the UNM HSC Facilities Planning Department for their continued support of the evolution of the library, especially Rick J. Henrard, Facility Planner, who has served as the primary architect for HSLIC projects since 1997; Stacy Kaneshige and Zoe Walton for the floor plan renderings; and former library associate directors Deborah Graham and Ruth Morris, who participated in Phase I planning.

Methods: A unique planning methodology was needed for a regular succession of projects to facilitate continuously evolving services and technology. Internal library teams were created to undertake planning and implementation. Planning and implementation methods were selected so that the library would remain open for use throughout renovations. Unlike many library renovations, the continuous improvement of the library facility depended upon internal funding and the work of an internal architect.

Results: Among the first outcomes of Phase I was the opening of an electronic classroom in January 1998. In addition, every collection item within public areas was relocated to accommodate new staff and service areas. Phase I was completed and celebrated when in 1999 the library served as the venue for the Health Sciences Center's Fifth Anniversary Celebration. Subsequent annual components of the project in Phases II and III have continued to accommodate new technologies. Data from user surveys conducted in 2002 and 2003 indicate user satisfaction.

Conclusion: This case study describes methodologies used to continually enhance the library facility in order to keep pace with programmatic changes and maintain high user satisfaction.

INTRODUCTION

Many publications detail new library building projects or one-time major renovations. This case study provides an overview of an ongoing process at the University of New Mexico Health Sciences Center (UNM HSC) to ensure the continuous improvement of library facilities. Shortly after the arrival of a new library director in the fall of 1997, the Vice President for Health Sciences at UNM announced an expanded role for the health sciences library. This expansion meant the creation of an academic and research technology development unit within the library. This new unit was intended to bring together librarians, information specialists, instructional technologists, and experts in computer sciences and multimedia to create, administer, and deliver information through the development of a collaborative structure. These initial programmatic and functional changes, consolidation of the HSC Computer Services with library services, and future developments required significant modification of the library's form and facilities. These changes were necessary to advance technologically and to respond to issues in a building that was too small for its expanded role.

Setting

The library was established as part of the School of Medicine (SOM) in 1963, in a building that was originally a soda bottling plant. Construction of the current library building started in 1975, and the facility opened to the UNM community in June 1977. The project was funded partially with a $2.24 million grant from the U. S. Department of Health, Education, and Welfare. The unique, award-winning, triangular-shaped building (see Figure 9.1) has two-story windows that face the Sandia Mountains (see Photo 9.1). The 65,800 gross square-foot building assigned approximately 40,000 net square feet to the library program on floors two through four. The first floor of the building was assigned to other HSC functions.

When the library building was constructed originally, its major user group was the SOM. In 1994, the HSC was officially formed by the UNM Board of Regents and was comprised of the SOM (including various allied health programs), College of Nursing, College of Pharmacy, five hospitals, and the library, which was designated as a freestanding academic component. By the mid-1990s, the HSC primary user group totaled approximately 6,000, including faculty, students, staff, and preceptors on campus and across the state. Therefore, an additional 3,920 square feet for remote storage for the collection was assigned in a building adjacent to the library building. (See Table 9.1 for a list of key service indicators measured since fiscal year 1996 (FY96).)

In 1997, it became apparent that a substantive addition, major renovation, or a new building was not immediately on the horizon for the library program. Subsequently, the HSC master plan published in 2001 projected needs for the library of at least 30,000 additional square feet, but an addition was not ranked for state funding until 2006-2007. However, discussions with the HSC Facilities Planning Department, along with approval from the Vice President's office to repurpose $300,000 of capital funding over three years suggested that

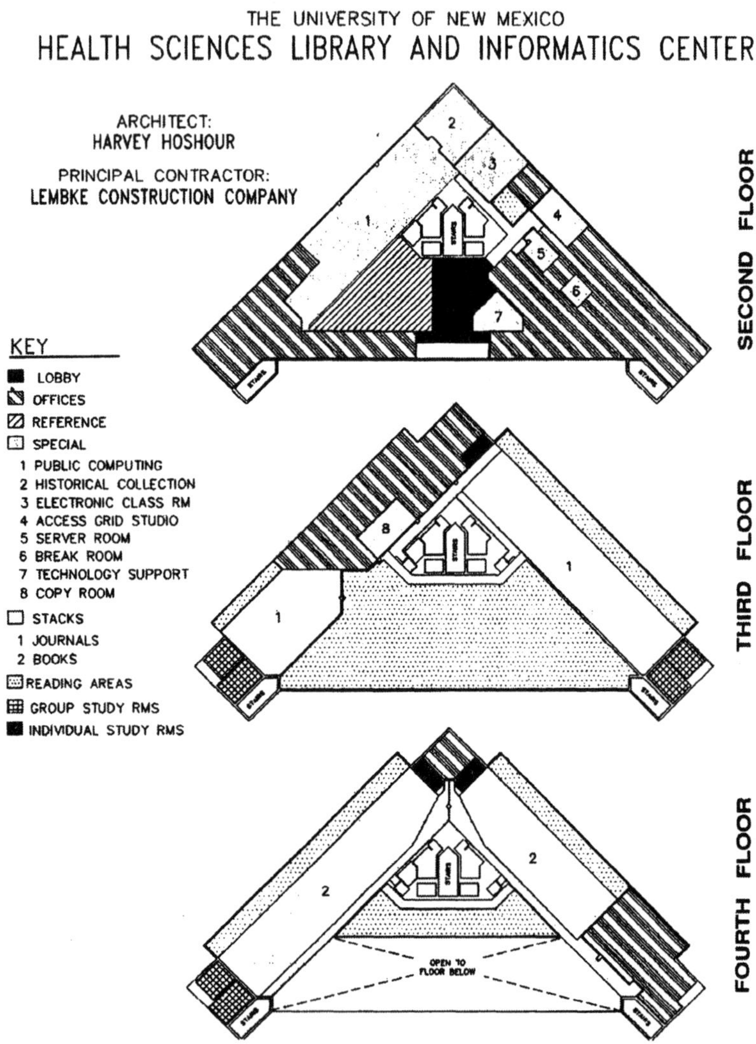

FIGURE 9.1. The library's unique triangular floor plan. Drawing by Stacy Kaneshige and Zoe Walton. Reprinted with permission.

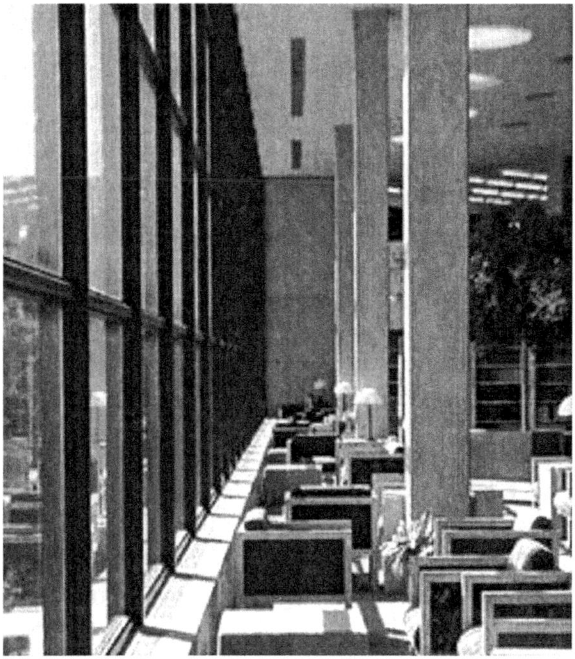

PHOTO 9.1. Reading area. Photo courtesy of David Groth.

TABLE 9.1. Service indicators, 1996-2003.

Service indicators	**FY1996**	**FY2000**	**FY2003**
FTEs	36.8	45.6	73.0
Gate count	252,940	263,841	314,068
Volumes	160,779	172,475	179,786

Source: Janis Teal.

an ongoing, annual process using funds from various sources, could sustain continuing renovation, provided that strategic thinking was done in advance and that library leadership remained aggressive in keeping the issue at the forefront of UNM leadership. Thus, a unique planning methodology was needed for a regular succession of projects to facilitate continuously evolving services and technology.

Objectives

As defined in its 1997 mission statement, the library assumed a critical role in creating a facility in which traditional library functions would be expanded to include interactive learning, technology-based education, and technology services. Phase I of the Library 2000 Project, as the remodeling project was known, identified and addressed several objectives critical to the library's transitioning to a role of technological responsibility within the Health Sciences Center. Several of the same objectives were further addressed in Phases II and III by subsequent remodeling projects.

By identifying existing problems and forecasting future needs, planners targeted several areas to be addressed initially. In 1997, public and instructional computing consisted of ten computers in the reference area and one 276 square-foot classroom that accommodated only seven students and that was not open for access other than during scheduled classes. The health sciences campus did not have a university computer pod. In a growing technological environment it was essential to provide for adequate computer-based instruction and to provide sufficient computers for curricular and productivity work. Achieving an increased role in technology was effected by moving HSC computer services into the organizational structure of the library and adding staff. The staff could double in the next five years, requiring a significant expansion of office space. Other workspace issues also needed to be addressed by relocating units and consolidating library service points to improve efficiency. The library's role in technology would require infrastructure upgrades to the network, power supply, and the server room; and the provision of technology-based conferencing in the library. An analysis of usage patterns of the collection demonstrated a need for improved ease of use. The current and bound journals were separated by two floors and photocopiers were positioned throughout the facility. When access was improved to collections, administrators learned that they also needed to improve collections security due to malfunctioning security gates.

Various other problems remained to be solved. The loss of a library staff lounge area to other HSC functions on the first floor of the building meant that staff would lose an amenity unless a new break room could be created in library-occupied space. Moreover, planners wanted the remodeling to create an aesthetically attractive environment where users would feel comfortable in accessing all resources, both technological and print.

Analysis of these problems resulted in the development of six objectives that would

- create facilities for instructional and public computing;
- create workspace to accommodate increased staff and to provide for increased efficiency;
- create a technology infrastructure capable of supporting the expanded role of the library;
- improve ease of use of the collection;
- improve security of the collection; and
- accomplish projects in such a way as to improve amenities for staff and users.

Although Phase I objectives (1997-1999) addressed strategic goals, Phase II (2000-2002) was characterized by more targeted, tactical objectives, addressing specific office space needs on the main floor as well as resolution of chronic plumbing problems in the twenty-five-year-old building, a strategy not funded until Phase III. Phase III objectives also were tactical: improving the workspace of off-site technology staff and the physical security of users in the library stacks. This case study will describe the three phases of renovation undertaken to achieve the six objectives (see Table 9.2).

METHODS

Soon after joining the University of Mexico in 1997, the director and two associate directors established the strategic planning group (SPG) with overall responsibility for ensuring a successful transition to a new physical and programmatic environment. Experiences gained by the director in an extensive strategic planning process at the Greenblatt Library at the Medical College of Georgia and knowledge gained from presentations at the National Library of Medicine's 1994 building symposium, "Building the Library/Information Center of

TABLE 9.2. Objectives, 1997-2003.

Objectives	Phase I (1997-1999)	Phase II (2000-2002)	Phase III (2003 and on)
1. Instructional and Public Computing	√		
2. Workspace	√	√	√
3. Technology Infrastructure	√		
4. Collection Access	√		
5. Security	√		√
6. Amenities	√		√

Source: Janis Teal.

the Future," which was published later as a special issue of *Computer Methods and Programs in Biomedicine,* provided the foundation for planning in New Mexico.[1] Other valuable resources included "The Technological Transformation of Health Sciences Libraries" by Newcomer,[2] and "Planning for Health Sciences Library Facilities" by Weise and Tooey.[3] In March 1998, internal library teams were created to undertake planning and implementation for the Library 2000 Project. Seven task forces were commissioned to focus on developing an organization for the twenty-first century: desk services; education services; staff development and training; serials/government documents/collection management; collection/archives; facilities; and systems. All staff served on one or more task forces. Unlike renovations in many libraries, the continuous improvement of the UNM HSC library facility has depended upon internal funding and the work of an internal architect. The project was also supported by the library's full-time position for both facilities management and purchasing functions.

As mentioned earlier, initial funding for Phase I was possible by repurposing three years of capital funding ($100,000 each year) to support renovation of the library, and by the assignment of an architect from the UNM HSC Facilities Planning department (Rick J. Henrard) to the project in 1998. Planning and implementation methods were selected so that the library would remain open for use throughout renovations, and Phase I was completed on schedule. Phases II and III have continued through the planning efforts of the strategic planning group (SPG), which has continued to meet monthly since its initial establishment. Ongoing funding has come from many internal and external sources. The 2002 creation of a new Administration/Informatics Suite on the fourth floor was partially funded by the Vice President's office with the condition that another HSC department temporarily use the space. UNM Physical Plant provided funding for carpeting and renovation of rest rooms to address ADA compliance issues. Grants from HRSA's Office for the Advancement of Telehealth, and the New Mexico state legislature provided funding to create videoconferencing facilities. Remaining projects have been funded internally by the library from salary savings from open positions or from contributions by other HSC components. Since 1997, over $1.3 million, excluding employee labor, has been invested in renovation and refurbishing the facility.

RESULTS

Phase I

Among the first outcomes of Phase I was the January 1998 opening of an electronic classroom. In addition, every collection item within public areas was relocated to accommodate new staff and service areas. Phase I culminated in a capstone event when the library was selected to serve as the venue for the Health Sciences Center's Fifth Anniversary Celebration in September 1999.

Instructional and Public Computing

Planners gave a high priority to developing a new electronic classroom that not only would expand instructional capacity but also would indicate the library's commitment to supporting all HSC academic programs, and not primarily the School of Medicine as formerly had been the case. Space in a separate building was used to create a twenty-workstation classroom and a multimedia instructional station. This classroom's use policy emphasizes its availability for curricular instruction by all instructors, not just librarian-educators, as well as a secondary purpose for noncurricular use. This classroom proved the ability of the library to plan and implement a major project benefiting all academic units of the HSC. It also paved the way for even more improvements, within the library building itself, the first of which was an additional twelve-station electronic classroom constructed in 1999. Because the HSC had no campus computing lab, the library's public computing area was expanded from ten reference stations to forty-eight stations that included curricular and productivity software. A small "multiuse development" (MUD) room was also created for special instructional needs.

Workspace

In 2000, one- and two-person offices in reference and user support services were fitted with modular units to accommodate two to four staff members. Modular offices were also created for technology staff in a second-floor area formerly occupied by collection resources. The information, circulation, and media service desks were consolidated into first two and then a single service point. Later, a small fourth-floor study room that housed the humanities collection became an office for accounting staff and the humanities collection moved to a smaller study room. In 2002, the computer help desk staff moved from their location in a separate building into library space formerly occupied by the media stacks. In 2003, the library obtained funding to renovate technology offices that remained in a separate building.

Technology Infrastructure

During Phase I, the library network was upgraded to a switched 100 Mb (megabit) network to the desktop in order to provide for increased Internet traffic from the public computing area, and the entire building received an electrical upgrade. In preparation for the growing technology responsibilities, planners upgraded the server room with a new heating, ventilating, and air-conditioning (HVAC) system. Through grant funding, a conference room constructed in 1997 was enhanced with studio lighting and equipped to become a studio on the Internet 2 Access Grid, enabling multicast conferencing—among the first fifty such studios in the country, and the first ever in a library.

Collection Access

In order to organize the collection more logically, the circulating books were moved to the fourth floor, and a formerly separate history of medicine collection (not the historical collection shown on the floor plan in Figure 9.1) was integrated into the circulating collection. Both the current journals and bound journals were relocated to the third floor, near a new photocopy room, where four copiers now provide more efficient and quieter copying. The new room features a glass wall into the hallway, making the area easily found by library users and alleviating fears of isolated users at night. Pre-1970 journals were moved to off-site storage, with paged access four to six times per day. The 1999 annual report announced, "A complete stack shift, including recarpeting and Americans with Disabilities Act (ADA) compliance, was completed in a record five weeks with no library closings."[4] By the time Phase I was completed, every collection item within public areas had been relocated to accommodate new staff and service areas and to improve functionality.

Security

In 2001, the library installed a new circulation security gate that used radio frequency (RF) technology. However, in 2002, the library returned to a more reliable technology by installing new electromagnetic security gates.

Amenities

A small kitchen/break room was constructed in the technology office area. New carpeting was installed on all three floors; complementary print and textured fabric was used on new chairs for the public computing area and to recover more than 300 existing club chairs used for studying. Benefiting from government purchasing rates, black mesh ergonomic chairs were purchased for the library classroom and conference room, as well as for staff offices. Of all the changes, these chairs best symbolized the forward-looking, modern new library. Providing a counterpoint to the high-tech nature of the remodeling, the Health Sciences Center helped the library to work with local artist Susan Linnell to display several large pieces. The artworks inspire interest and comment in a visually harmonious environment. Subsequent project components continue to accommodate new technologies.

Phase II

In Phase II, the consolidation of computer services and library services into the new Health Sciences Library and Informatics Center (HSLIC) required additional new office space to accommodate administrative needs and two new faculty positions related to informatics and education development. A new administrative suite was designed and built on the fourth floor, incorporating two study rooms.

Phase III

In 2003, physical plant funds became available to remodel the rest rooms on the second floor, in a project that was completed in early 2004. Unstable shelving units and security incidents in the stacks led to funds at the end of fiscal year 2003 being targeted for a video surveillance system throughout the facility and for stack braces (tie struts) to anchor all full-height stacks not previously secured.

Future Plans

Six years of remodeling (1997-2003) resulted in the library's becoming a symbol of the Health Sciences Center's entry into the world of advanced technology. New offices were created for the manager of special collections and distance librarians; a "stop-and-drop" area was built in the technology office area for quick computer access by off-site staff; and collection resources workflow was reassessed in light of the electronic era. The two existing electronic classrooms will be complemented by two mobile classrooms accommodating an additional twenty-eight students.

USER SURVEY

Additional information was gleaned from user surveys administered to library patrons. By conducting an internally developed survey of users in 2002 and by participating in the LibQUAL+ survey in

2003, the library was able to gain statistical feedback about the variable, "Library As Place" (to borrow a concept from the LibQUAL+ survey). The 2002 Web-based survey obtained results from 498 respondents. Two of the twelve questionnaire items related to the "Library As Place," workstation availability, and study rooms. On a five-point Likert scale, the mean score of all respondents for workstation availability was 4.02, among the highest item means. The mean score for study rooms was 3.41, the lowest item mean.

A survey question asking "What is the best thing about the library?" received 338 responses and mentioned the following physical-environmental features (listed in decreasing order by number of comments):

- Computers
- The general environment
- Quiet/noise
- Study rooms
- The view

Actual comments testified that the library is a "great place to study," and mentioned view of the mountains from the reading area. In response to the 2002 survey question, "What is the one thing you would change about the library?" 352 responses were received, and the following physical-environmental features received mention:

- Study
- HVAC system
- Computers
- Quiet/noise
- Environment

The 2003 LibQUAL+ survey, with 307 respondents, gave high marks to HSLIC on the "Library As Place" dimension, with an adequacy mean of 1.07 and a superiority mean of –0.40, both better than the library's overall adequacy mean of 0.80 and superiority mean of –0.66. Scoring for individual items in the "Library As Place" dimension is shown in Table 9.3. For benchmarking comparison, the adequacy mean and superiority mean for all of the Association of Academic Health Science Libraries (AAHSL) participating in the

TABLE 9.3. HSLIC and AAHSL scoring for "Library As Place" dimension LibQUAL+, 2003.

Item	HSLIC adequacy mean[a]	AAHSL adequacy mean	HSLIC superiority mean	AAHSL superiority mean
Quiet space for individual activities	0.93	0.48	−0.48	−0.81
A comfortable and inviting location	1.52	0.76	−0.06	−0.71
Library space that inspires study and learning	0.99	0.43	−0.62	−0.97
Community space for group learning and group study	0.93	0.55	−0.51	−0.79
A getaway for study, learning, or research	1.01	0.54	−0.44	−0.81

Source: Janis Teal.

[a]By assessing the minimum level of acceptability to users, desired level, and actual (perceived) level, LibQUAL+ results allow the calculation of an "adequacy mean" (perceived score minus acceptable score) and a "superiority mean" (perceived score minus desired score). Higher scores are better on both the adequacy mean and the superiority mean, although even a good superiority mean is frequently a negative number.

LibQUAL+ survey are also shown. UNM HSLIC scored above the mean for all AAHSL libraries on all items in the "Library As Place" dimension. In addition, HSLIC scored above the mean for all Association of Research Libraries (ARL) respondents with the exception of one item: "Community space for group learning and group study."

The 234 comments received on the LibQUAL+ survey paralleled the 2002 internal survey comments, including wanting more study rooms, quieter environment, and more effective HVAC. Positive comments included the following:

- "I appreciate the comfortable chairs and spaces to learn."
- "The view of the mountains from the third floor makes spending a day inside studying not so sad!"
- "The HSC library is well-organized, conveniently located, and I could not ask for a more helpful, knowledgeable, and courteous staff."

Critical comments mentioned the "disappearing group study rooms," suggested "some space modification to allow for better individual study and group learning," and requested "more study areas with tables and less lounge-type chairs."

CONCLUSION

This case study has overviewed the methodologies used by the UNM Health Sciences Library and Informatics Center to continually enhance the library facility to keep pace with programmatic changes and maintain high user satisfaction. Based on experiences since 1997, the authors can identify several lessons learned and affirmations about the planning process.

First, although major efforts were undertaken to add new formal, group learning space (electronic classrooms and conference rooms), user survey respondents stated that they wanted more space that "promotes human interactivity" where people can "gather and think together in a casual way." The relationship of communities of practice to knowledge exchange is increasingly recognized as applicable for library environments, as evidenced by articles in *Information Outlook* and the virtual continuing education seminar given by the Special Libraries Association in January 2004.[5-7] As a result of remodeling and repurposing study rooms for staff offices and workspace, the original number of group study rooms was reduced from nine to six. A study room reservation system is available for scheduling rooms, but only 11 percent of available room time was scheduled in advance. The library promotes the system as a way to improve availability of rooms to students. Library leadership will continue to explore creative ways of providing various types of space to support communities of practice, within the constraints of existing space.

Second, should the library have to plan future renovations, earlier planning and proactive training for consolidating three service desks into a single service point would have reduced renovation and staffing costs incurred by making multiple moves.

Third, the MUD room was not well-utilized. Although the planners expected faculty to make computer assignments that could be completed in the MUD room, these assignments were not forthcoming, and the MUD room may have been an idea before its time.

Fourth, the HVAC system dates to the construction of the building, and while routine HVAC assessments have been conducted, the physical plant department recognizes that this area needs improvement.

Fifth, through knowledge gained of the university facility planning process, the remodeling project grew into an opportunity to participate in campus-wide information technology planning that resulted in the development of UNM-wide IT infrastructure standards for new and renovated buildings.

Sixth, the security gate replacement experience taught the library staff that sometimes early adoption of new technology has unexpected results, even for technological leaders on campus.

Last, regardless of the lessons learned, it is possible to initiate and sustain renovations over a long period of time resulting in substantive changes, given ready access to in-house facilities planning expertise and the involvement of library staff. Ongoing renovation has proven to be a good strategy. Until the master plan evolves to make a library addition possible, this methodology will assure that the library facility continues to be responsive to user and staff needs, and leverage changes in programs and technology.

NOTES

1. Ball, Marion J., Weise, Frieda O., Freiburger, Gary A., and Douglas, Judith V. (Eds.). "Building the Library/Information Center of the Future." *Computer Methods and Programs in Biomedicine* 44(September 1994): 141-270.

2. Newcomer, Audrey Powderly. "The Technological Transformation of Health Sciences Libraries." In *Administration and Management in Health Sciences Libraries,* Rick B. Forsman (Ed.). Lanham, MD: Medical Library Association and The Scarecrow Press, 2000.

3. Weise, Frieda O. and Tooey, Mary Joan. "Planning for Health Sciences Library Facilities." In *Administration and Management in Health Sciences Libraries,* Rick B. Forsman (Ed.). Lanham, MD: Medical Library Association and The Scarecrow Press, 2000.

4. Buchanan, Holly Shipp. *Annual Report FY 1998/99 Executive Summary.* Available online at <http://hsc.unm.edu/library/annrept/annrep699.cfm>.

5. Lee, James and Valderrama, Kathy. "OPS's Are Networks of Activities." *Information Outlook* 7(May 2003): 18-23.

6. Abram, Stephen. "Communities: The Three R's—Roles, Relevance, and Respect." *Information Outlook* 7(June 2003): 25-28.

7. Wallace, Deb and Pauloski, Linda. "Building Communities of Practice for Knowledge Exchange." Special Libraries Association Virtual Seminar (January 23, 2004).

Case Study 10

The McGoogan Library of Medicine: A Value-Added Approach to Renovation

Nancy N. Woelfl
Stuart K. Dayton
Tom Gensichen
Mary E. Helms
Marie Reidelbach

OVERVIEW

Setting: The McGoogan Library of Medicine is an academic health sciences library that serves the University of Nebraska Medical Center (UNMC), its teaching hospital, and the state of Nebraska. The three-story structure opened in 1970. By 1995, the building was in urgent need of renovation.

Objectives: A sustained planning process secured a $2 million state allocation to accomplish four major objectives:

- Rewire and install network connections at study seats on two floors.
- Redesign and significantly improve the lighting.
- Replace carpets and wall coverings.
- Reconfigure and relocate customer service points.

Methods: The renovation was guided by a number of principles: a library should be a premier information service, not a storage facility; new construction or added library space were not

The authors acknowledge Rod Cope, Head of Circulation, and Steve Bridges, Library Assistant, for their exceptional and tireless efforts throughout the renovation as well as colleagues and co-workers who contributed toward successful completion of this project.

needed; and the importance of getting the most out of every project dollar. Construction began in October 1999 and was completed in December 2000. Although it was not business as usual, the library operated continuously throughout the fourteen-month renovation. High levels of formal and informal communication were essential throughout the project.

Results: An area measuring 41,811 square feet was renovated at a cost of $47.85 per square foot. Construction costs totaled $34.35 per square foot. Primary colors of red and black were replaced with a teal, blue, and ecru color scheme, maple wood finishes, curved surfaces, and accent lighting. Laptops can now be used in all renovated areas. The lighting redesign was successful. All furnishings and seating were replaced; and a networked user lounge with vending machines was added. Exit surveys of graduates indicate high satisfaction with the library.

Conclusions: Given the difficulty of financing new construction, the McGoogan Library is a prime example of what can be done with existing space. The project team was able to address both infrastructure and aesthetic issues on a constrained budget. Staff contributed services allowed the library to save thousands of dollars. The structure makes a visible statement about UNMC's belief in the value of library services.

INTRODUCTION

Setting

The Leon S. McGoogan Library of Medicine is a three-story, 58,629 gross square-foot academic health sciences library that serves UNMC, its 735-bed teaching hospital, the state, and region. Opened in 1970, the library building approached the end of its planned life cycle by 1995. The electrical and telecommunications systems were inadequate for distributing increasing amounts of electronic information and shelves were filled to almost 95 percent of capacity.

The library lobby is built around a freestanding staircase backed by a three-story mural of the DNA helix. During the 1980s, the circulation and reserve desks were combined and moved into the middle of the lobby, surrounded by public photocopy machines (see Photo

10.1). The circulation desk presented a fortress-like appearance to arriving users. Although staff were customer friendly, they stood with their backs to the door. The reference area was relatively open and barrier-free, but customers had to navigate a tangle of wires to get to the desk. Six workstations stood atop the old card catalog in a position that was ergonomically awkward for users. Natural light from corner windows reached some areas of the interior but most illumination came from coffered ceiling lights. The coffers, located fourteen feet above the floor, illuminated only the top two shelves of stacks and delivered even less light to work surfaces.

The effects of heavy use were apparent throughout the library. The carpeting was worn through to the subfloor and taped with duct tape where it could no longer be patched. Although the library worked diligently to incorporate new technologies, workstations were concentrated in the few areas that could be easily wired and networked. Not only was the McGoogan Library an increasingly uncomfortable place to work, it was ill-equipped for a digital future. By 1995 the library began to surface regularly in student surveys as a source of dissatisfaction.

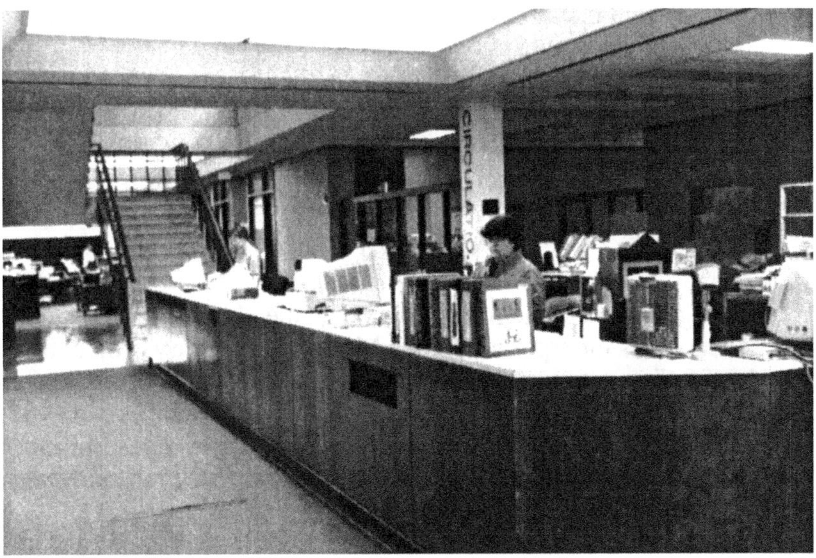

PHOTO 10.1. The circulation desk stood in the middle of the lobby. Photo courtesy of the McGoogan Library of Medicine. Used with permission.

Objectives

A new library building was not an option for UNMC, nor was one needed. As the transition to electronic full text gained momentum, the staff was confident that existing space was sufficient for the library's needs. This case study describes the assumptions and construction processes that transformed the library from a depreciated facility nearing the end of its life cycle into an inviting venue that will not only serve UNMC for years to come but incorporates features and amenities valued by users of all types.[1-3]

The process that secured renovation funding involved hard work, careful planning, and occasionally, a little luck. More than ten years elapsed from the start of the library's space planning process to the onset of construction. In 1996, the Nebraska Legislature passed a bill authorizing $97 million in deferred maintenance spending for the University of Nebraska system, including a $2 million allocation for the McGoogan Library. The renovation program statement released in January 1997 outlined four major objectives:

- Rewire and install network connections at all study seats on the sixth and seventh floors.
- Redesign and significantly improve the lighting.
- Replace carpets and wall coverings.
- Relocate major service points in proximity to the entrance.

METHODS

Although it took some time to verbalize the phrase "value-added," the concept was incorporated in the McGoogan Library project from the day funding was announced. Based on a building consultant's report, the cost of total renovation was estimated at $5,121,500 in 1992, and the library was advised to escalate the estimate by 4 percent every year construction was deferred. Using this base, a total renovation would have cost $6,739,000 by 1999.

Funding academic construction has never been easy and is becoming increasingly difficult.[4] The staff understood a state allocation of any amount was an affirmation of the library's value and resolved to get the maximum benefit out of every project dollar.

"Sizing" the scope of construction to the budget required some difficult decisions. Because renovating all three floors on a $2 million budget was out of the question, the library decided to concentrate on levels six and seven, the two floors that would make the biggest difference to users. Renovation was an ideal time to replace the HVAC control system, but these repairs were deferred. Students badly needed a user lounge, but construction would have to wait for a private donor. The library waived competitive selection of an architect and relied on a campus architect with previous library design experience, saving thousands of dollars in fees and expenses that were channeled into the building. By agreeing to pack and shift the collection, the library staff helped ensure additional thousands were conserved for capital equipment instead of being spent on temporary labor. Finally, in anticipation of renovation, the library accumulated unrestricted endowment income in a reserve fund, knowing there would be unanticipated expenses.

The architect made frequent visits to the library, probing functional problems in each area scheduled for renovation. He then produced five concept drawings that began to put a face on the "new" library. One of these images generated a major gift toward the cost of the user lounge. Detailed floor plans for the sixth and seventh floors were developed and are shown in Figures 10.1 and 10.2. Original floor plans are shown in Figures 10.3 and 10.4. Whereas simple enhancements were planned for level seven, the sixth floor was significantly changed. An Omaha engineering firm designed mechanical and electrical systems for the building and prepared the blueprints used by the general contractor and subcontractors.

PROJECT PHASING

Each rectangular floor of the McGoogan Library measures 110-feet wide by 200-feet long and is approximately 20,000-feet square in size. The construction plan developed by the general contractor divided the work into four ninety-day phases, for a total planned construction time of twelve months. Each ninety-day phase targeted half a floor, approximately 25 percent of the total space to be renovated. Closing the library for even a portion of the renovation was not an option. Phasing allowed both the general contractor and the library to

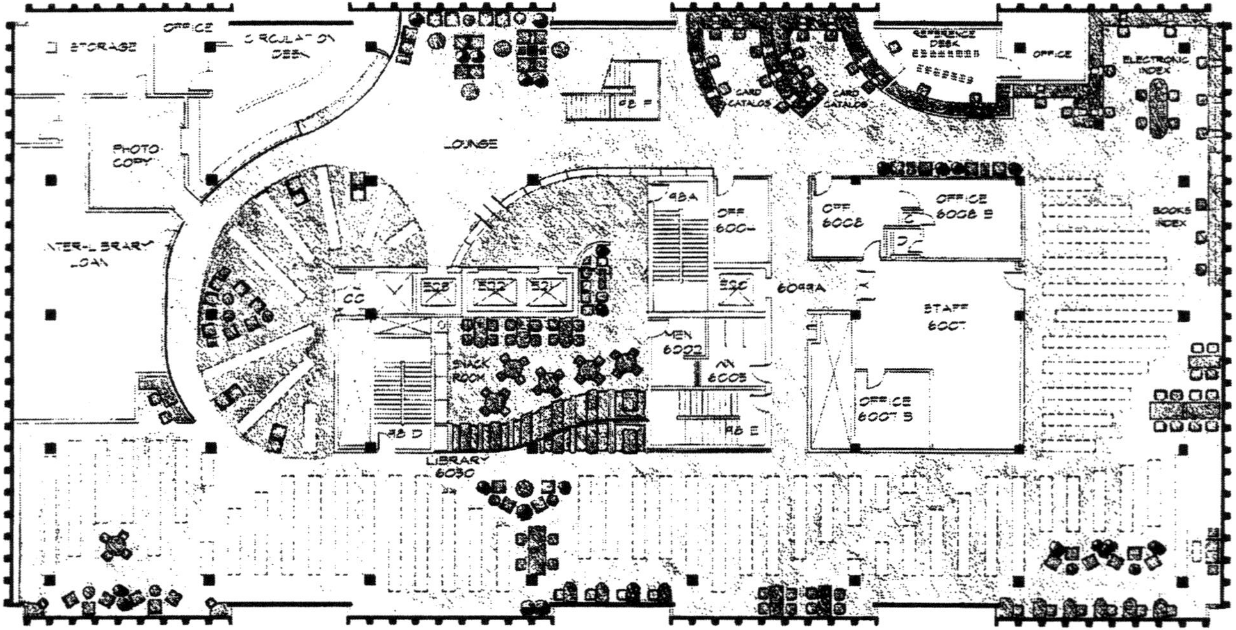

FIGURE 10.1. Detailed floor plans for sixth floor. Courtesy of McGoogan Library of Medicine. Used with permission.

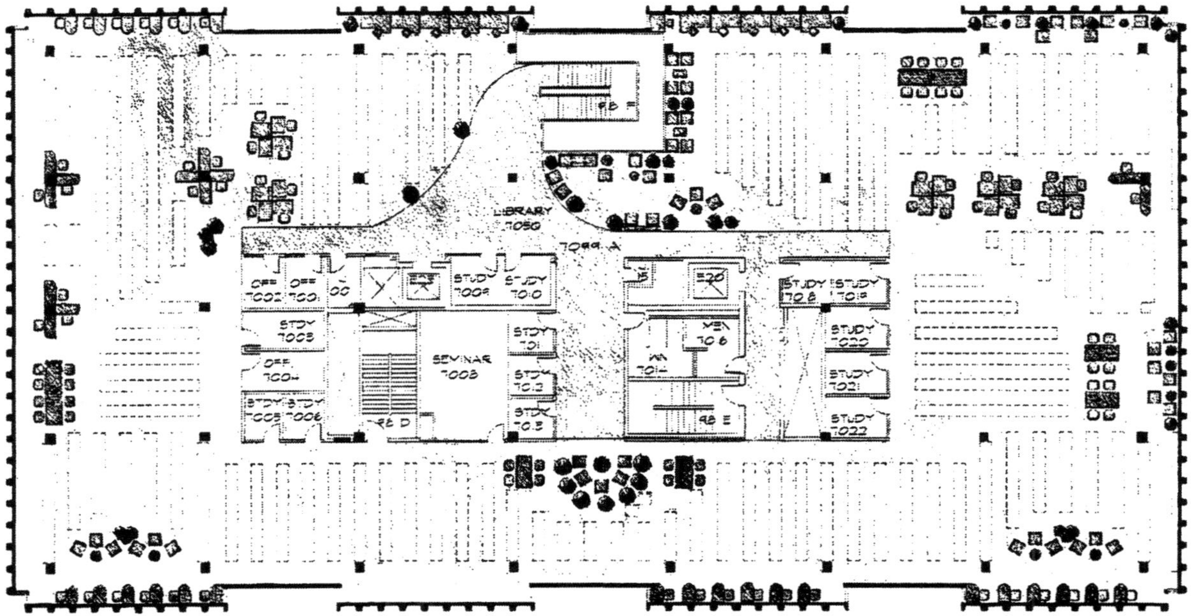

FIGURE 10.2. Detailed floor plans for seventh floor. Courtesy of McGoogan Library of Medicine. Used with permission.

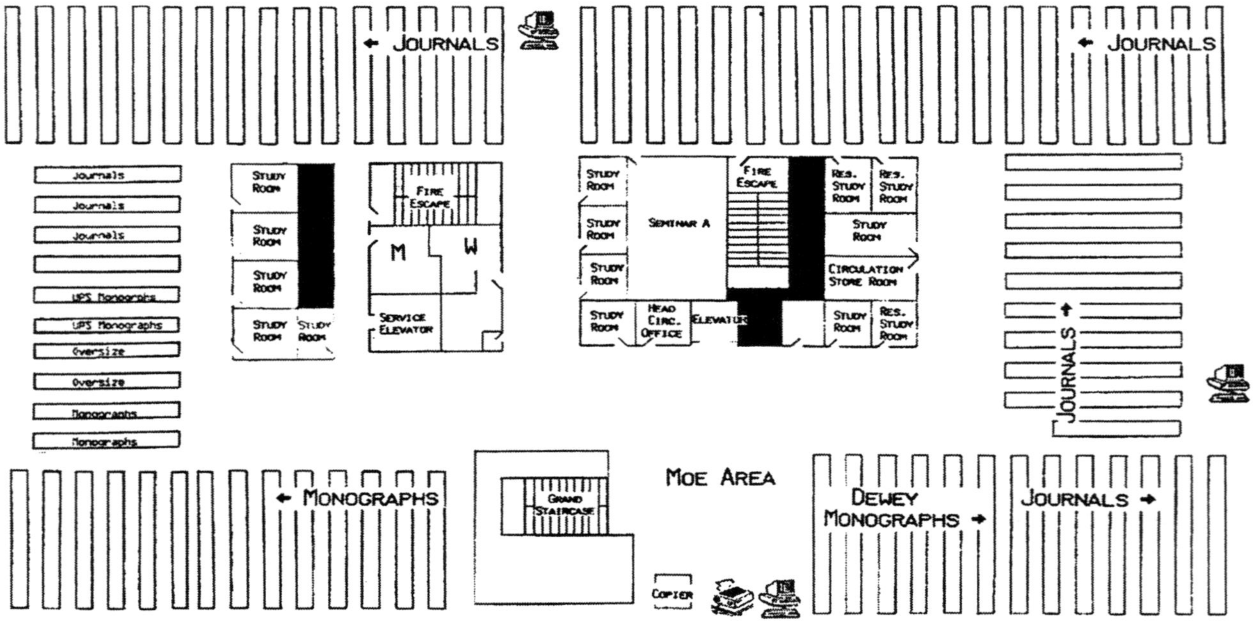

FIGURE 10.3. Illustration of sixth-floor layout before renovation. Courtesy of McGoogan Library of Medicine. Used with permission.

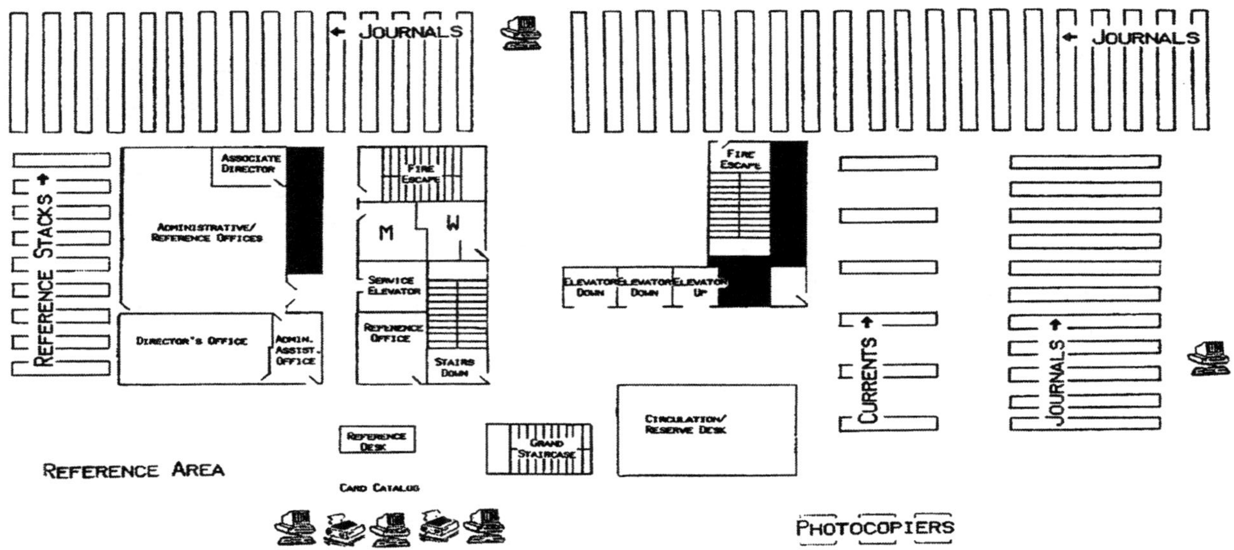

FIGURE 10.4. Illustration of seventh-floor layout before renovation. Courtesy of McGoogan Library of Medicine. Used with permission.

operate in the building simultaneously. Phase 1 concentrated on constructing new service points at the north end of the sixth floor. Phase 2 focused on new reference and reading areas at the south end. Phases 3 and 4 involved the north and south halves of the seventh floor respectively. The general contractor prepared a detailed timeline for each phase.

Downsizing and Moving the Collection

Before Phase 1 could begin, the library had to move at least 20 percent of the collection out of the building to create space for construction equipment and supplies.

Floor plans for the new shelf configuration were used to calculate how many linear feet of shelving would be lost and how many would remain for books, journals, and reference material. Every shelf that would be permanently removed was conspicuously tagged, along with its contents.

Circulation statistics and focus group results were used to size the collection to the remaining shelf space and allow some room for growth. Focus groups indicated faculty did not rely on volume counts as a quality indicator and were more concerned that the library function as a premier information service. Based on this input, ceased titles unrelated to active subscriptions, state medical journals, and nineteenth-century French, German, and Italian language titles were targeted for temporary or permanent removal. Location changes were entered in the online catalog, with off-site volumes designated as "not available for use."

From July through September 1999, library staff packed almost thirty tons of material. Using a reader lounge on the sixth floor as a staging area, they filled and accumulated boxes for transfer to the storage site, a vacant building owned by UNMC Facilities Management. The boxes were labeled with color-coded content lists to ensure redelivery to the appropriate library level after construction or holding in storage until exchanged, sold, or recycled. Materials removed from the shelves filled 1,000 boxes weighing approximately sixty pounds each. Less than 50 percent of this material returned to the shelves after construction.

Surplus shelves were dismantled. Using a stack mover leased from the Lincoln City Libraries, professional movers eased fully loaded shelves into the configuration designed by the architect. The shelves and their contents were then covered in seamless plastic sheets and taped at the corners. In all, the library staff shifted the journal collection five times during the renovation and shifted the book collection four times.

Living with Construction

Construction began on October 19, 1999. Although library operations continued throughout the project, it was not business as usual. Noise, collection access, maintaining telephone and network connections, delays in phasing, and drywall dust took a toll on users and staff alike. Intensive communication was essential throughout each phase of the work.

There was no way to avoid noise, especially at the start of each construction phase. As each successive area was gutted to the shell, slabs of falling sheet metal shook the library and the offices below it. Construction workers were constantly reminded to keep their voices down. The sound of concrete drilling and stud nailing set teeth on edge throughout the building.

As much as possible, demolition work was scheduled from 6:00 a.m. to noon, when students were in class. The academic calendar was checked to ensure that noisy tasks did not begin the day before major examinations. A quiet study area was established on the eighth floor and prominently posted signs directed students to it.

Maintaining collection access during what turned out to be fourteen months of construction was difficult. Twenty-five percent of the journal collection was behind construction barriers during Phase 1. The remaining journals and book collection were out of reach during Phases 2, 3, and 4.

To maintain access to the most current literature, active journals published in 1998 and 1999 were shelved in a public area adjacent to the new circulation desk and a retrieval service was established to pull volumes behind construction barriers. Users submitted forms at the circulation desk; requests submitted by 3:30 p.m. Monday through Friday were ready for pickup after 9:00 a.m. the following morning. The library operates with minimal weekend staff, so requests submitted on Saturday or Sunday were usually held until Monday morning, which was a source of frustration for requestors. Unclaimed items were reshelved after twenty-four hours, which also led to friction between the desk staff and users.

All staff participated in the retrieval service on a rotating basis but the work quickly became tedious due to dust, lack of lighting, and the plastic shelf coverings. At the start of Phase 3, the head of circulation and another long-term staff member offered to accept sole responsibility for pulling and reshelving user requests. Both worked sixteen-hour days during the last two phases and received overtime pay for their Herculean efforts. From October 1999 through July 2000 at least 16,000 items were pulled and delivered to users. Monthly statistics ranged from a low of 681 to a high of 4,439, with an average of about 1,350 volumes per month.

Maintaining telephone and network connections throughout construction required careful planning, communication, and coordination. Close working relationships between the library and campus information systems departments played a key role in ensuring that staff in areas under construction had uninterrupted telephone and data connections throughout the process. As one area neared completion and the next was about to begin, the library delivered detailed checklists of telephone extensions and datalines to be moved, and tested them afterward to make sure they were live. Frequent walk-throughs of construction areas were essential to check actual installations against blueprints, and to request reinstallation if incorrect. During construction, the systems department operated under the mantra "plan, talk, walk, and look."

Project Delays

Despite careful planning and good project management, delays occurred during every phase of the project. Although the staff can look back and laugh, most of these problems were not funny at the time. The first was related to the stack lighting, which though not elaborately designed, could not be securely mounted to the stacks. The redesign delayed parts production and when manufacturing began, it took several weeks of trial and error to refine finishing techniques. Anticipating slack time, a local auto body shop planned to spray paint the fixtures but had a hard time supplying the parts when their repair business picked up unexpectedly.

Lighting installation got back on track only to have another delay. To avoid carpet damage, carpet installation was scheduled as the last task in every phase. As the first phase drew to a close, the flooring subcontractor tried to substitute inferior carpeting for the product specified in his proposal. This dispute almost reached the point of litigation.

The importance of being able to interpret blueprints, visualize the results, and understand their functional implications was reinforced on many occasions. By the time it became apparent the reference desk would measure forty-eight inches from floor to top, the metal studs shaping the curved console had already been installed (see Photo 10.2). To eliminate a customer service barrier, the service stations were widened and the marble countertop notched to allow the librarian to come forward toward the user. On the customer side, the marble was extended to create a toe space, bringing the user closer to the librarian. By installing swivel screen monitors, both could work at a mutually comfortable distance to review and refine search results.

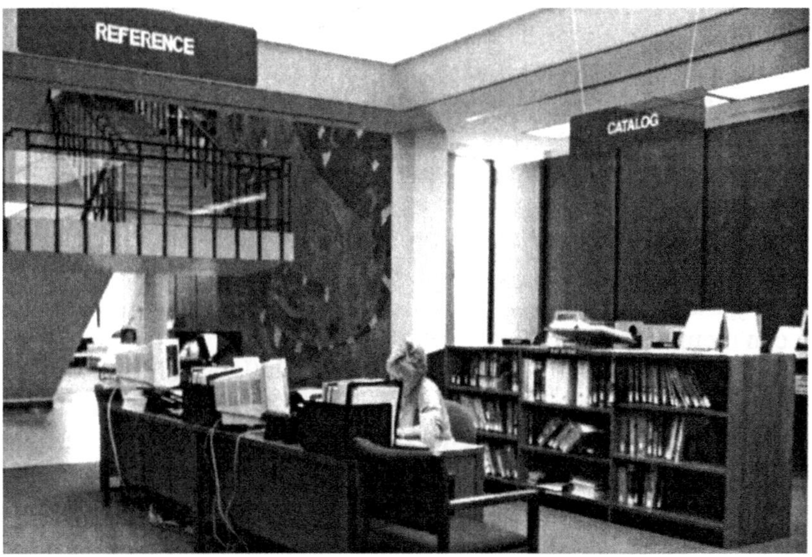

PHOTO 10.2. The old reference desk was cramped and inefficient. Photo courtesy of the McGoogan Library of Medicine. Used with permission.

Although noise was a stressor, it was also a sign of progress. One Monday morning during Phase 3, the day began with unwelcome silence. Level seven had been painted the previous week and this work was scheduled to continue. Painters, however, were nowhere to be seen and did not return for almost three weeks because of a local strike.

After months of construction, the third and fourth phases were not routine because some of the most intricate construction work was left for last, including curved-glass walls and bookcases in the lobby. In addition, as unfinished space dwindled, the remaining construction supplies were consolidated in the lobby, creating a visual eyesore in the midst of the nearly completed structure.

Dust Control

The previously described problems paled in comparison to dust control, the single most costly and demoralizing problem of the entire renovation. From the beginning, the library emphasized dust containment and protection of the collection as paramount responsibilities of the general contractor. It was understood some dust was inevitable, but nothing prepared the library staff for hours of backbreaking work that resulted from ineffective dust-containment practices.

The general contractor used a number of measures to control plaster dust. These included thick construction barriers with a minimum of doors; ventilating equipment that maintained negative air pressure inside the construction area; and sweeping or vacuum cleaning at the end of every shift. When dust accumulated on the sixth floor shelves during the first two phases, the library used endowment income to clean them commercially.

By the time Phase 3 started on the seventh floor, retrieval service had been underway for more than seven months, with the pull rate basically doubling each month. Interlibrary loan staff also continued to pull and reshelve, adding to the wear and tear on the tape and plastic coverings. The adhesive tape failed and without a tight seal, the plastic sheeting lost most of its protective value. The drywall subcontractors on the seventh floor also refused to sweep, vacuum, or follow dust-containment procedures and intentionally provoked conflicts with the project foreman. When the drywall workers departed, they left a quarter inch of drywall dust behind, but there were no funds left for commercial cleaning.

After expressing anger and frustration, library staff rolled up their sleeves and went to work. UNMC Environmental Services delivered cases of treated cloths so shelves and printed material could be dry-dusted. Although dust masks proved uncomfortable and were soon abandoned, latex gloves were essential and worn at all times. The director insisted on and received cleaning assistance from the general contractor but by the time it arrived, the library staff had finished most of the work. The seventh floor contained more than 3,000 linear feet of shelving. Cleaning shelves and the materials on them were as physically taxing as packing.

FORMAL AND INFORMAL COMMUNICATION

Coordinating complex renovation processes required intense levels of formal and informal communication. On-the-spot consultations about work in progress took place daily. A construction coordinating committee met weekly to review the project status, exchange information, and resolve problems. The minutes of this meeting, compiled by the general contractor, proved to be one of the most valuable communication tools of the entire process. These minutes were circulated widely, posted in the staff lounge, and excerpted for various publications, including the library Web page. Keeping staff in the loop helped improve morale by providing staff with the information needed to serve customers and answer questions. Humor also played an important role in maintaining morale. The staff produced a video patterned on *The Blair Witch Project,* a 1999 horror film. The staff video hinted to construction workers that the library was haunted, showing pictures of a shadowy, ethereal Dr. McGoogan peering between the wall studs with a faint but approving smile on his face.

RESULTS

With the exception of the user lounge, construction work was completed in December 2000. An area measuring 41,811 square feet was renovated at a cost of $2,393,200. The final project budget is shown in Table 10.1. Decisions to exceed state allocation were carefully justified and offset using contingency funds, endowment income, and gifts. A UNMC donor contributed $100,000 toward lounge construction that totaled $173,000 (see Photo 10.3).

TABLE 10.1. McGoogan Library of Medicine final cost accounting, June 30, 2001.

Expense	Total cost
Design coordination	
a. In-house architectural/engineering services	$71,500
b. Outside architectural/engineering services	125,000
c. Project supervision	38,500
d. Reimbursable expenses	5,000
Construction contracts	1,286,000
Movable equipment	314,000
Insurance	10,000
Contingency	150,000
Lighting and ceiling upgrades	118,916
Study carrels with electric power	19,864
Flooring at entryway	15,414
Study room improvements	5,252
Conference room renovation	
a. Computer	3,436
b. Projector/smart board	11,792
c. Construction contracts	19,864
User lounge	
a. Display wall	31,935
b. Ice maker	3,127
c. Furnishings	7,413
d. Construction contracts	130,527
Shelving	6,881
Signage	9,455
Cleaning	9,326
Total	$2,393,202

Source: Nancy N. Woelfl.

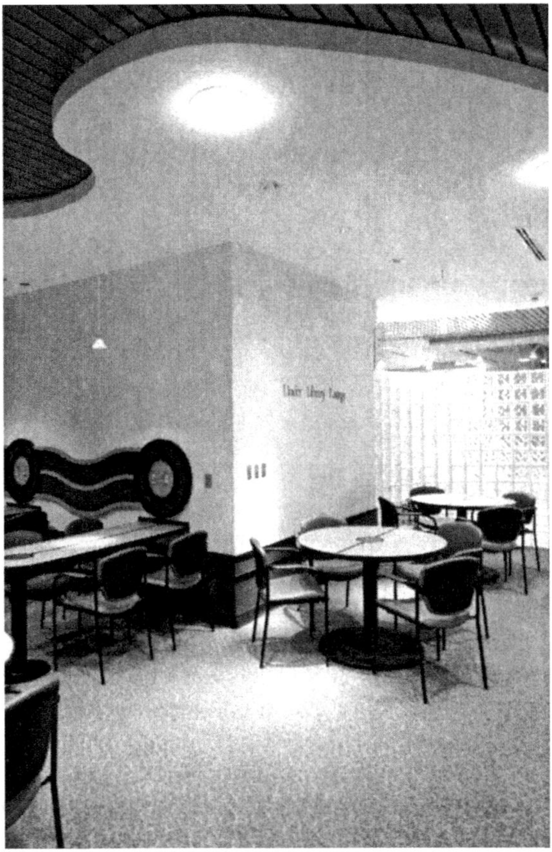

PHOTO 10.3. The user lounge features network connections and vending machines. Photo courtesy of Schemmer Associates, Omaha, Nebraska. Used with permission.

In 2001, Richard Bazillion described six qualities of a value-added academic library and the infrastructure needed to evoke them. He noted that "in many cases buildings of 30 years old or more simply cannot be renovated to suit today's information environment, at a cost most institutions can bear. They have to be replaced."[5] The McGoogan Library is one of the exceptions to Bazillion's observation.

As each successive section of the building was gutted, new electrical and telecommunications wiring was installed in all public and staff areas. Transaction-intensive areas such as circulation, reference, and interlibrary loan operate at 100 Mb over Ethernet cable. Ten lounge booths, public, and staff workstations operate at 10 Mb. Seventy-five study carrels along the walls and around interior structural columns are also wired for power and 10 Mb Ethernet service.

Wireless Networking

Prior to the renovation, the library explored the possibility of installing a totally wireless network but the campus infrastructure was not yet ready to support this technology. The renovation significantly increased network connections for laptops and other portable devices and laid the foundation for a postrenovation wireless network.

Lighting

By the end of the renovation, lighting had gone from being the most frequent complaint to the most frequently cited library improvement. Although there was no increase in natural light reaching the interior, a significant improvement was made in the quality of light inside the structure. Architect John Howard noted a desire for libraries that emphasize natural light and "transparency," qualities that characterize the renovated McGoogan Library despite its concrete shell.[6]

Most lighting was removed from the ceiling and lowered to the work surface. Each study carrel has an individually controlled work light; table lamps are wired through floor chases and channeled up through each table. Top-bracketed stack lights illuminate all six shelves instead of the top two. A lighted, glass block wall transfused by softly glowing colors separates the user lounge from the library entrance and illuminates the ceilings above circulation and reference.

Interlibrary loan moved from the eighth floor to the northeast corner of the sixth floor, adjacent to circulation, in a place that customers can easily find. A public photocopy room is located between the two departments; all three service points are interconnected via a room that doubles as a locker/paper storage room. Course reserves and circulation supplies are concealed behind visual screens that keep physical and visual clutter out of the lobby. The lobby was transformed into an open, inviting space with enough room to house the library's consumer health collection on shelves just inside the door. It is easier for patients and Nebraska residents unfamiliar with the library to find materials and nearby staff are available to assist them.

Two stand-alone reference desks were replaced by a built-in console with a continuous marble countertop. The curved twenty-seven-foot console features two service stations and a modified work area for persons with disabilities. An elevated facade conceals search tools. Reference handouts and supplies are organized in pigeon holes located between the two service bays (see Photo 10.4).

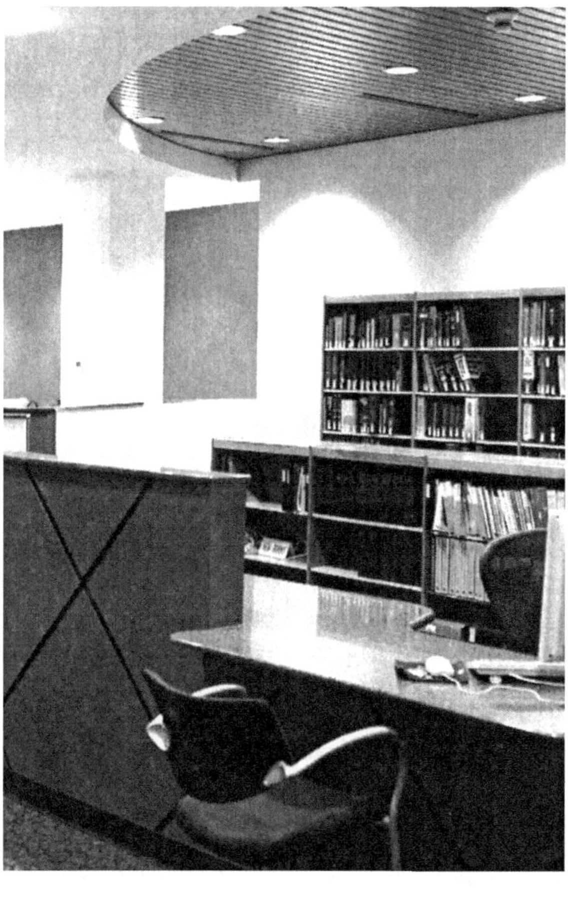

PHOTO 10.4. The new reference desk is staff- and user-friendly. Photo courtesy of Schrader-Marcus Photographics, Lincoln, Nebraska. Used with permission.

Sixteen end-user workstations occupy two U-shaped configurations behind a sixty-inch facade that separates them from the lobby. Continuous countertops provide comfortable distance between workstations and enough room to spread out notebooks, reference materials, and papers. The partition between the bays was lowered to forty-eight inches, allowing customers to make eye contact with a librarian. Recessed lighting minimizes screen glare on the workstation monitors.

Furnishings and Decor

From the beginning, the library worked to create a space that reflected the professional roles of its primary-user constituency. Managing to address aesthetic issues and infrastructure on a constrained budget is another reason the McGoogan Library project can be considered a value-added renovation.

The architect worked with an interior designer to develop a color palette that coordinated the carpets with wall coverings, furnishings, and woodwork. Their design services saved time and made the number of color choices manageable. Shades of slate blue, teal, and ecru unify the interior without being dark or heavy. Two different carpet patterns were used: deep navy with splashes of beige in high traffic areas and muted blue with a subdued paisley background in office and study areas. Wood paneling was replaced with painted drywall that has diamond-shaped cuts in the surface to eliminate long, monotonous walls.

Although tables remain, there are fewer of them. Over time, the library staff observed a consistent pattern of one user per table, with strangers reluctant to share space with someone they did not know. Students also avoided the original study carrels, which seated four in an efficient spokelike configuration. As a result, the library replaced multiple seat units with as much single seating as possible, even though this resulted in some seat loss. New tables and study carrels feature birch and maple laminated surfaces (see Photo 10.5).

Product catalogs were used to identify institutional-grade furnishings that could meet student expectations for comfort without collapsing under hard use. Chairs with flexible metal frames, sled bases, and plastic parts that allowed the seating to "breathe" were selected. The seating subcontractor provided samples for users to try out and the test introduced an element of fun into the renovation process. It

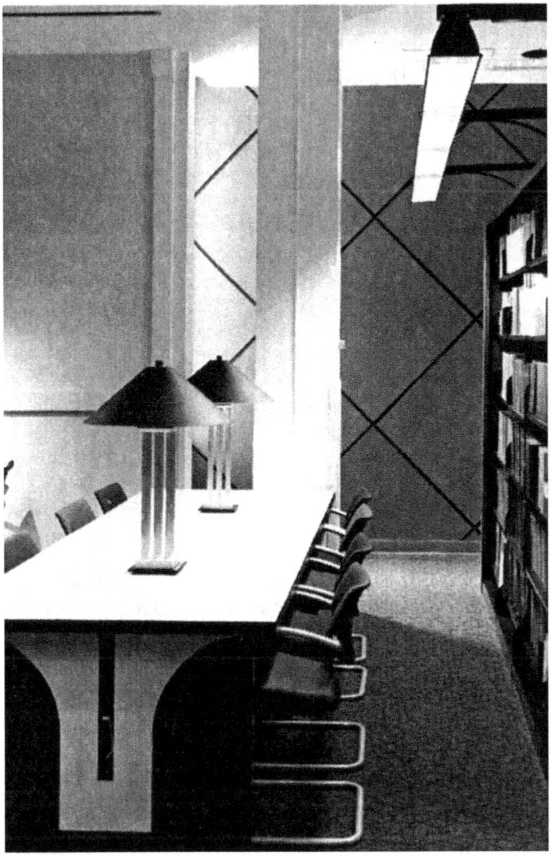

PHOTO 10.5. Study area lighting, seating, and woodwork. Photo courtesy of Schrader-Marcus Photographics, Lincoln, Nebraska. Used with permission.

also helped provide assurance user preferences would be taken seriously when seating was ordered.

The library purchased 260 units of new seating, upholstered in shades of blue, rust, and cream. Several different types of study chair were ordered to give users a choice. New chairs were purchased for some of the staff. Leather club chairs were placed in the lobby (see Photo 10.6). Upholstered easy chairs and three large couches are tucked away in quiet reading areas. Sixteen recliners are among the most appreciated pieces of furniture in the library.[7]

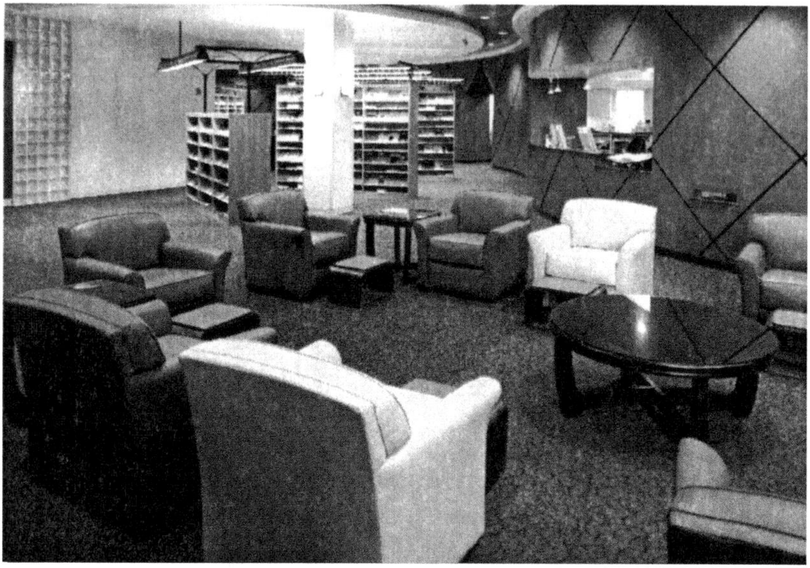

PHOTO 10.6. McGoogan Library lobby and circulation area. Photo courtesy of Schrader-Marcus Photographics, Lincoln, Nebraska. Used with permission.

LESSONS LEARNED

The McGoogan Library offers lessons for other libraries contemplating or scheduling a large-scale renovation. The first and most important lesson is the need to plan carefully and budget for dust control. Renovation projects should contain a specific line item for commercial cleaning. Even though the general contractor used current industry practices, these practices do not work effectively in occupied buildings. Limited cleaning done when Phase 4 was still in progress was a poor investment of money. The library should also have done a better job of documenting subcontractor misconduct and insisting offending companies or personnel be removed from the job.

Libraries planning totally new buildings are most likely to benefit from competitive architectural selection, but those planning renovations should consider local firms. Functionally and aesthetically, McGoogan Library outcomes were excellent due to the amount of time the architect spent on-site prior to and during renovation. Fee and expense savings were an added bonus.

Master blueprints should be revised to reflect changes that are made during construction and saved along with other working documents. Photographs should be taken to document before, during, and after views of construction. Without them, location details related to wiring and cabling are quickly forgotten.

The McGoogan Library sent some withdrawn materials into storage to avoid the public relations nightmare that may occur when users or the public see bound volumes in dumpsters. Recycling or discarding publications is difficult but should be done immediately. Moving these volumes consumed funds that could have been used for other renovation-related purposes.

CONCLUSION

The renovation ended officially with an open house on October 11, 2001. As guests gathered on UNMC Alumni Day, all who had a role in the process were publicly acknowledged. The renovation was one of the most difficult yet rewarding tasks the library staff has ever performed, requiring discipline, teamwork, and the ability to meet seemingly impossible deadlines. But in a profession where tangible outcomes are not always visible, everyone who took part could see what his or her work accomplished.

User comments indicate a high degree of satisfaction with the renovation. The project received an award from the American Society of Interior Design.[8] The McGoogan Library regularly hosts visits from building consultants and other librarians planning space improvements. The library was pictured in *American Libraries* and has been the subject of local news coverage.[9] A recent Association of American Medical Colleges (AAMC) survey of graduating medical students indicates student satisfaction with the library has improved (see Photo 10.7). Fifty percent of UNMC medical students graduating in 2003 indicated that they were very satisfied with the library. In contrast, only 35 percent of 2001 graduates gave the library this score. The Class of 2001 not only saw the library at its prerenovation worst, but they also lived through the renovation as third- and fourth-year students.

In terms of cost per square foot, the McGoogan renovation was extremely cost efficient. Excluding the user lounge, the construction

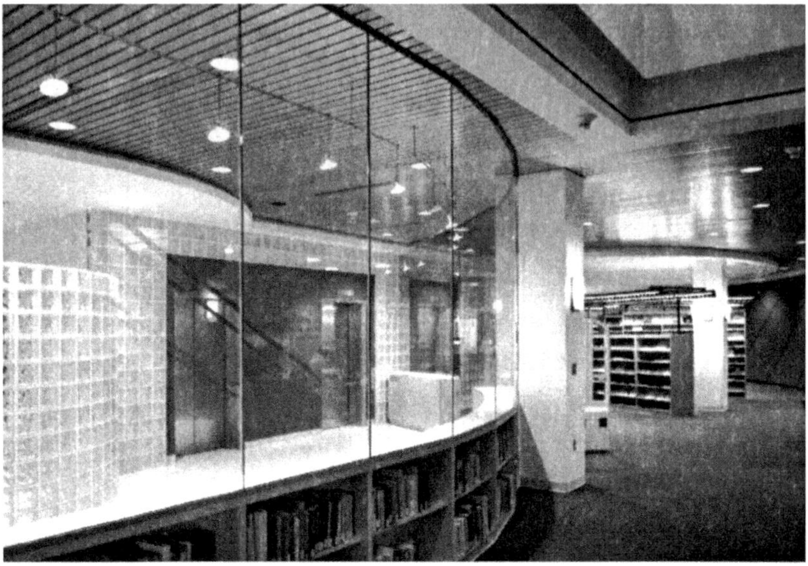

PHOTO 10.7. A transparent lobby invites users in. Photo courtesy of Schrader-Marcus Photographics, Lincoln, Nebraska. Used with permission.

cost per square foot equaled $34.35. Factoring in administrative overhead, contingency, and fees, the project total was $47.85 per square foot. A sampling of comparable projects completed in 2000 shows renovation costs ranging from $14 to $134 per square foot, with an average of $58.45.[10]

The McGoogan Library renovation project was successful for a number of reasons. The project was comparable to larger institutional values. The library understood the financial and political realities and did not ask for or expect the impossible. The renovation was justified in terms of documented user needs and problems, particularly the library's deficiencies as a learning environment and student facility. The project also had numerous advocates. Students frequently discussed the library with the Chancellor and occasionally the Board of Regents. Faculty continued to affirm the links between the library, curriculum, and the cultivation of lifelong learning skills in students.

Although some project efficiencies are related to lower construction costs in the Midwest, contributed staff services comprise the greatest value-added input to the renovation process. Staff willingness to perform strenuous tasks that could not be budgeted, particularly post-construction cleaning, allowed the state to acquire more construction goods and services than would otherwise have been possible for $2 million. Their voluntary services during the renovation were an extension of stewardship they have shown toward the McGoogan Library building for many years and an extraordinary gift to the University of Nebraska Medical Center and the people of Nebraska.

NOTES

1. Kenney, Brian. "The Library Reloaded." *School Library Journal* 49(December 2003): 8-10.
2. Albanese, Andrew Richard. "Deserted No More." *Library Journal* 128(April 15, 2003): 34-36.
3. Burke, Linda. "The Saving Grace of Library Space." *American Libraries* 35(April 2004): 74-76.
4. Shill, Harold B. and Tonner, Shawn. "Creating a Better Place: Physical Improvements in Academic Libraries 1995-2002." *College and Research Libraries* 64(November 2003): 431-466.
5. Bazillion, Richard J. "Academic Libraries in the Digital Revolution." *Educause Quarterly* 24(2001): 51-55.
6. Kenney, "The Library Reloaded," p. 9.
7. Olson, Jeremy. "Med School Students Find Comfy Sofas and Recliners." *Omaha World-Herald* (January 17, 2001): 13, 16.
8. Stansberry, Rhonda. "It's All in the Design: Midlands Interior Designers Are Recognized for Excellence at an Annual Competition." *Omaha World-Herald* (June 24, 2001): 10E.
9. "Foundations of Knowledge: Libraries Realize Their Vision of Room to Grow." *American Libraries* 32(April 2001): 56.
10. Fox, Bette-Lee. "Strength in Numbers." *Library Journal* 125(December 2000): 50-61.

Case Study 11

Ebling Library: Planning a Three-Library Merger and Move

Sylvia Contreras
Erika Sevetson
Natalie Norcross
Julie Schneider
Daniel Barkey

OVERVIEW

Setting: The University of Wisconsin (UW)–Madison Health Sciences Libraries (Power Pharmaceutical Library, Weston Clinical Science Center Library, and Middleton Health Sciences Library) were merged into a new facility, Ebling Library, in June 2004. The new library includes a technologically supported learning environment with wireless network capability on all library floors, multimedia/digital lab, and patron seating capacity of over 350. A single service desk combines the reference and circulation areas of each library.

Objective: To merge and move the collections and staff of three libraries into one new library facility.

Methods: Four key planning committees were established: public relations, service integration, information technology, and collection shelving and preparation. Committee responsibilities included ensuring internal and external communication of building project information; examining the implications of merging three service desks; determining the technological needs of the library, designing multimedia use strategy, and identifying technologically related building integration issues; assessing and consolidating three physical collections;

and developing a process to minimize the transfer of clutter to the new facility. Each committee utilized the library's intranet to post agendas, documents, and other related material.

Results/conclusions: The committee structure was successful. Committees developed timelines, information fact sheets, frequently asked questions (FAQs), and a collection-assessment process; and identified core service desk skills and staffing levels. A strong communications network alleviated some of the stress associated with planning a merger and move of this size.

INTRODUCTION

The Health Sciences Libraries (Power Pharmaceutical Library, Weston Clinical Science Center Library, and Middleton Health Sciences Library) at the University of Wisconsin–Madison merged into a new facility. During planning phases, the building was referred to as the Health Sciences Learning Center (HSLC) Library; it is now known as the Ebling Library. The new library is the heart of the multidisciplinary educational facility, serving the needs of all health sciences schools, programs, and centers. In bringing scattered resources together, the library provides comprehensive health information services and access to a world-class collection.

The approximately 50,000 square-foot Ebling Library includes a technologically supported learning environment with wireless network capability on all library floors, nineteen research workstations, eighteen-seat library education room, multimedia/digital lab, sixteen group study rooms, and seating for more than 350 patrons. A single service desk combines the current reference and circulation areas of each library.

The approximately 160,600 usable square-foot building (approximately 255,000 square-foot gross) consists of two wings: a three-story, crescent-shaped, north wing and a four-story south wing. A central atrium connects all of the above-grade floors. Learning facilities include a 350-seat auditorium; one 60-seat, one 110-seat, and two 175-seat lecture halls; and other education and retail spaces.

History of the Project

The west side of the UW campus was designed to enrich the multidisciplinary needs of all health science schools, programs, and centers. Major west side construction initiatives began with the signing of HealthStar legislation (1997), a six-year state and university partnership to construct a School of Pharmacy facility, interdisciplinary research complex, health sciences learning center, utilities, and replacement parking facilities.[1] The project was jointly funded through state and university sources. Groundbreaking on the HealthStar initiative began in 1998, with construction of the School of Pharmacy facility.

During initial stages of HSLC building planning, a request for proposal (RFP) was developed by the medical school administration and other health science administrators. After much review, the Kahler/Slater architectural firm was selected to design the Health Sciences Learning Center project. Kahler/Slater and the UW Facilities Planning and Management Group established the following focus groups composed of future HSLC occupants: Library Resources, Study and Instructional Resources, Technology Core, Administrative Core, and Building Services Core. These user group meetings were held regularly. Each member was encouraged to participate in brainstorming and evaluation sessions. Construction guidelines and constraints were provided to each group. In addition, Kahler/Slater provided the library with a consultant. The consultant met with each library unit to discuss the specific spatial and design requirements of that unit. The Library Resources core group provided the architects with a list of requested design features, including unit adjacency requirements, adequate space provision for individual staff workstations, a single service desk centering around a "one-stop shopping" model to meet both information and circulation needs, and a spacious and comfortable learning environment. Kahler/Slater then presented the various user groups with the first draft of the building design. Each user group was given the opportunity to comment on the drawings, discuss the design concept, and suggest modifications (see Figures 11.1, 11.2, and 11.3).

When the design was completed and construction began, staff of the Health Sciences Libraries started planning the move and merger

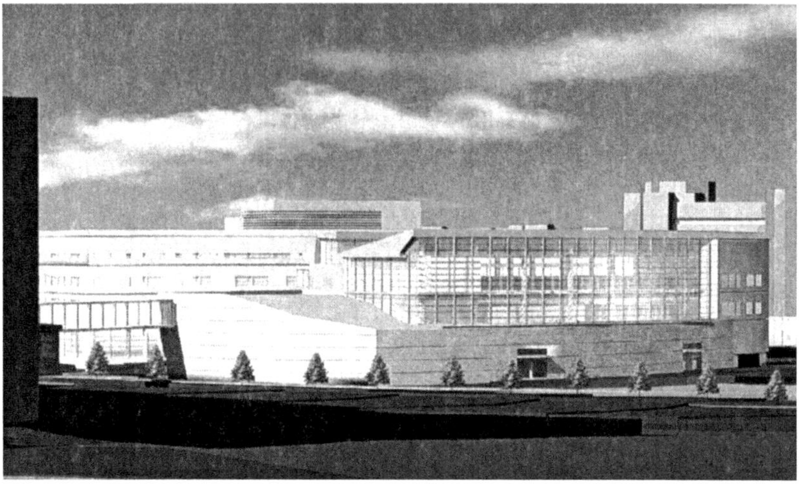

FIGURE 11.1. Architectural exterior rendering, northern view.

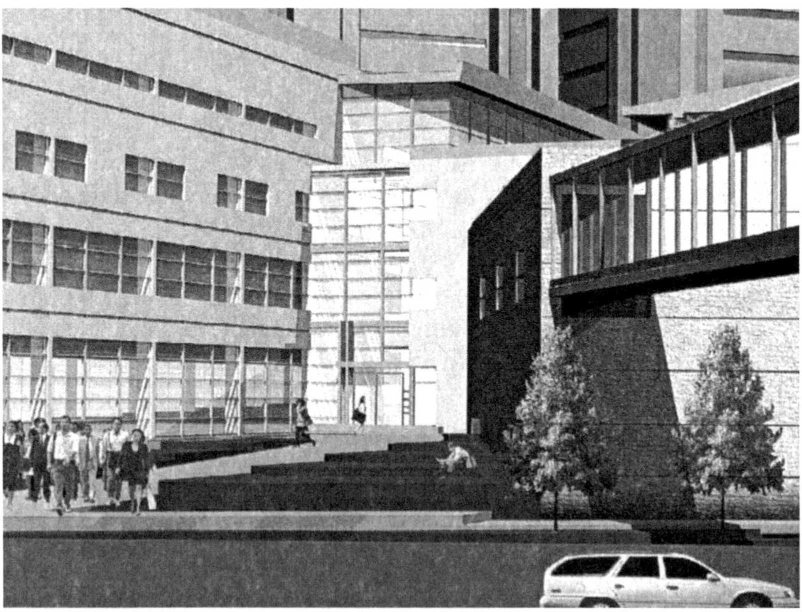

FIGURE 11.2. Architectural exterior rendering, front entrance.

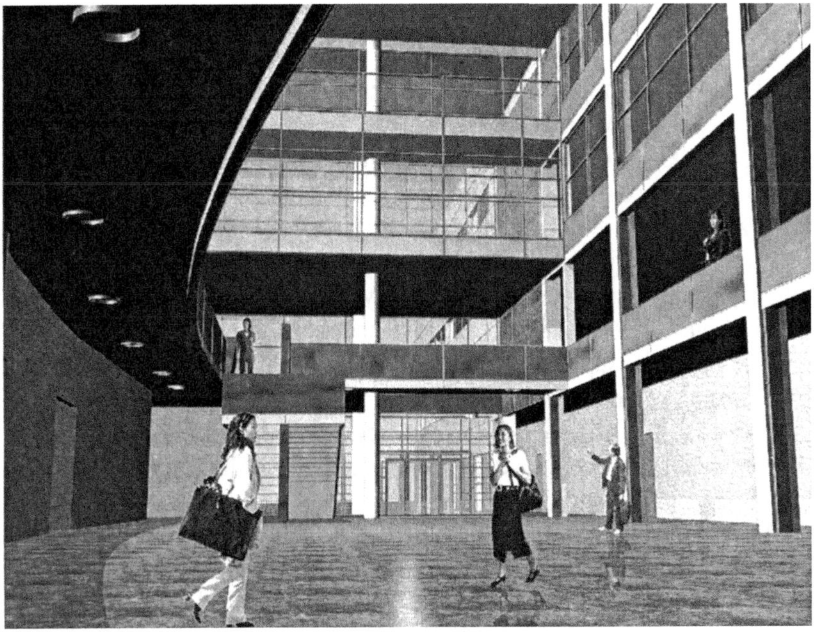

FIGURE 11.3. Architectural exterior rendering, atrium.

of the three libraries. Four key planning committees were formed: service integration, collection shelving and preparation, public relations, and information technology.

Library planning committees were charged with examining the implications associated with the merger of four library service desks in three buildings; planning for the merger of the collections and staff of three libraries into one new facility; assessing and consolidating four physical collections (including a collection in storage); determining the technological needs of the library, designing multimedia use strategy, and identifying technologically related building integration issues; ensuring that information regarding the building project was communicated both internally and externally; and developing a process to minimize the transfer of clutter to the new facility. Each committee completed a literature review and utilized the library intranet to post agendas, documents, and other related material.

SERVICE INTEGRATION

The service integration committee examined the various implications associated with combining library areas and merging multiple service desks. A list of action items was brainstormed and prioritized and used as a road map for the work of the committee. Work began with a multistep exercise of imagining the approach to the new service desk from the patrons' point of view, determining the needs of entering patrons, and visualizing how library staff would work together behind the desk to meet those needs. In an effort to standardize service statistics collection as much as possible and gain an overview of current use and trends, an inventory was taken of current service statistics kept at all three libraries. A common service philosophy for the entire library was drafted, discussed with all departments, and adopted as the business standard.

Another focus of the committee was to determine the appropriate staffing necessary at the service desk. Smaller working groups met to discuss an hourly staffing plan and skill sets needed by each type of staff. Traditionally, library services assistants (LSAs) have worked at circulation desks and professional librarians have worked at reference desks. Therefore, combining the physical desks to create "one-stop shopping" for patrons necessitated an integration plan for staff duties. A detailed list was developed to describe the core skills necessary to assist users. Discussion of who should do what at the service desk continued among staff in many forums over several months, and was guided by library administration's view that hand offs of patrons should be minimal and that the patron would ultimately decide whom to approach with questions. The basic-skills requirement would likely expand to include more reference knowledge by LSAs and more circulation knowledge by librarians. Although staff envisioned reference and circulation experts at different ends of the desk during peak hours, they needed to work as a team at all times. Administration broadened the skills list to encompass fundamental knowledge and skills required of all library staff. Planning of staff training skills was transferred to the staff training and development committee. Additional work of the service integration committee included identifying staff equipment needs, consolidating telephone numbers without using telephone trees, and determining how to meet patron needs on the second floor of the library, where the only service area is within the History of the Health Sciences collection.

Using a multidisciplinary committee to identify service needs of patrons and training needs of staff allowed a common vision to evolve naturally with input from all staff. The time taken to let ideas percolate was time well-spent in preparation for such a major shift in operations.

COLLECTION SHELVING AND PREPARATION

In the early stages of planning new library facilities, much time is spent measuring and determining current and future space needs of collections and staff. With careful calculations, estimates can be made for growth and potential changes to the collection over a preselected number of years. When the final decisions are made on building layout, the most difficult part of the planning and preparation process for collections is just beginning.

The collection shelving and preparation committee ensured the assessment and move preparation of all materials in the three collections. In addition, the committee developed an appropriate shelving floor plan for the new library, coordinated and trained the selected moving company, and organized all collection-related move issues.

The committee began its work by looking at the current status of the collections and compiling the following information:

- Formats of the collections
- Locations of the collections (physically and in the OPAC)
- Moveability of materials
- Size of each part of the collections
- Cataloging used for each part of the collections

Following this information-gathering exercise, the committee worked out a tentative list of individual projects and a timeline of completion for each. Because the collections were spread among three libraries and one storage location, the committee focused on identifying any major difficulties.

From the outset, the committee realized that the journal collection would take the largest amount of preparation work and would involve many of the staff in all three libraries. The three biggest obstacles to preparing the journal collection were the number of volumes of journals not yet bound, number of volumes duplicated among the three libraries and other campus libraries, and the fact that the journal collections were arranged in three different organizational schemes.

Since a decision had to be made on a single organizational scheme for all journals, the committee spent considerable time identifying the advantages and disadvantages of various plans. That information was then shared with all library staff, opinions were collected, and library administration decided that the journal collection in the new building would be organized by the classification system used in the main library collection. In addition to assessment of the journal collection and identification of duplicate volumes, the committee created a plan for reclassifying the journal collections at two of the locations, relabeling each volume, and shifting the collections into the same classification scheme. Work on the journal collection consumed nearly 80 percent of the committee's time, took the most planning, and also required the most communication with the entire library staff.

Additional work of the committee included preparing the rest of the collections for the move, measuring all parts by location, determining shelving needs in the new building including estimates for growth, developing a shelving plan, and communicating all collection changes to library staff.

INFORMATION TECHNOLOGY

The information technology planning committee determined the technological needs of the library, designed multimedia use strategy, identified new positions, and identified technologically related building integration issues. The greatest challenge for this committee was projecting needs three to five years in advance, a process that approximates crystal ball gazing.

In the early stages of information technology (IT) planning sessions, library operations and services were planned separately from the rest of the building occupants. Although the classrooms and teaching labs would be used to deliver content and to educate students using a state-of-the-art visual network, the library would be the place to develop content and systems to organize and provide access to a vast store of knowledge.

As the building developed into a technologically advanced facility, the various IT groups in the Medical School, School of Nursing, and libraries merged together into one building-wide unit. The newly merged library information technology group attempted to define the building IT infrastructure, considered new ways to utilize technology, planned loosely for new technologies, determined IT staffing levels, determined building-wide staff equipment needs, and designed a collaborative multimedia/digital lab.

During initial planning stages, the library information technology group focused on creating the Multimedia/Digital Lab, which was physically and operationally attached to the Library Systems department. The design concept centered around the theory that content creators, IT staff, and librarians would collaborate on technology-based initiatives. As the concept developed, several key design elements were identified. The lab would have a small user resource library, offer several high-end workstations with a vast array of multimedia equipment and software, be located within the library to enhance collaboration with librarians and IT staff, and offer a small conference room for group collaboration.

Infrastructure planning centered on providing wireless network capabilities in most public areas of the building. Although the library would continue to place research workstations along the entrance, patrons would not otherwise be exposed to the physical characteristics of technology. The open network jack would be replaced by all-encompassing wireless access, and students would connect to the network from anywhere in the building, no longer restricted to the physical location of the network connection.

PUBLIC RELATIONS

The public relations committee ensured that information regarding the project was communicated internally to all staff and externally to users and other campus libraries. The first task of the committee was the development of the project Web site, which served as the primary external communication vehicle. The site included the "Health Sciences Learning Center on the Move 2004" logo and links to news and updates, fact sheet, project overview, FAQs, construction images, floor plans, and construction updates.

Web-site development included brainstorming sessions to determine which information required mass distribution. Using this process, the project Fact Sheet was developed, providing basic information regarding the construction project, including library features and services, overall building and library square footage, building occupants, project funding, and associated project costs. The FAQs generated by staff, faculty, and students was another communication vehicle that emerged from the brainstorming sessions. The committee also developed the "Health Sciences Learning Center on the Move 2004—Ask Me" button, which library staff wore to promote awareness of the project and stimulate discussion between library staff and users.

CLUTTER ERADICATION

In order to move three libraries efficiently and to minimize the transfer of clutter from existing facilities to the new facility, a kiss it good-bye subcommittee was formed to develop a clutter eradication plan, assist staff in organizing their offices, and consolidate the files of three existing libraries. The office organization plan was based on the FlyLady Home Organizational System and the Kiss It Goodbye Campaign developed by the University of North Carolina, Chapel Hill.[2-3] Staff enhanced the record-retention policy, created an archives-retention policy, developed office zones, and established weekly decluttering missions. Staff were encouraged to weed their work-areas, paper files, electronic files (e-mail and other documents), and personal belongings for fifteen minutes per day. The daily sessions allowed staff to take incremental steps toward achieving a clutter-free environment and establishing routines. Units were assigned a weeding representative to assist staff with the weeding, archiving, and recycling process. Progress included the removal of over 2,500 pounds of material, identification and future removal of dated furniture and equipment, and awareness of a useful office-organization system. Collaborative and individual efforts were strongly encouraged and rewarded.

The committee also worked on a major marketing campaign to promote the new facility and services. The committee met with campus publicity departments to design a new marketing strategy, worked with a design consultant to develop a new logo, and developed key sound bites for staff to share with users.

CONCLUSION

Planning for a three-library merger was challenging and rewarding. Staff participated in all levels of planning, proposed excellent ideas, and brought those ideas to fruition. A strong communications network alleviated some of the stress associated with planning a merger and move of this size. The most challenging aspects of the construction project centered around the formulation of a technology plan; evaluation, assessment, and weeding of the collections; and communication to staff and users throughout all phases of the project. Physically integrating the collections in an efficient and effective manner were also challenging. Communications about minimal service and closure were developed and distributed to all identified user groups.

As the building took shape and became the true point of integration for the health science schools, the library was poised to meet the challenges and needs of the interdisciplinary group. The effectiveness of the planning processes depended on how well the library's vision met the university's vision of interdisciplinary collaboration.

NOTES

1. "HealthStar: Facilities and Programs for the 21st Century." *Quarterly: The Wisconsin Medical Alumni Magazine* (winter 1998): 12.
2. Cilley, Marly. *Sink Reflections: FlyLady's BabyStep Guide to Overcoming CHAOS*. New York: Bantam Books, 2002. Available online at <FlyLady.net>.
3. University of North Carolina, Kiss It Goodbye Campaign.

RECOMMENDED READING

Cirillo, Susan E. and Danford, Robert E. *Library Buildings, Equipment, and the ADA: Compliance Issues and Solutions*. Chicago: American Library Association, 1996.

Dancik, Deborah Bloomfield. *Building Blocks for Library Space: Functional Guidelines*. Chicago: American Library Association, 1995.

Hagloch, Susan B. *Library Building Projects: Tips for Survival.* Englewood, CO: Libraries Unlimited, Inc., 1994.

McCarthy, Richard C. *Designing Better Libraries: Selecting and Working with Building Professionals.* Fort Atkinson, WI: Highsmith Press, 1995.

Metcalf, Keyes D. *Planning Academic and Research Library Buildings.* Chicago: American Library Association, 1986.

Michaels, Andrea A. and Michaels, David L. *Interior Design and Furniture Selection for Libraries.* Scottsdale, AZ: Michaels Associates Design Consultants, Inc., 1998.

Sannwald, William M. *Checklist of Library Building Design Considerations,* Third Edition. Chicago: American Library Association, 1997.

Case Study 12

The Welch Medical Library: A New Model for the Delivery of Library Services

Willard F. Bryant Jr.
Jayne M. Campbell
Kathleen Burr Oliver
Nancy K. Roderer

OVERVIEW

Setting: The William H. Welch Medical Library of the Johns Hopkins University in Baltimore, Maryland, is the focal point of the planning development activities described in this case study. The authors will describe the results of a master planning effort depicting the library of 2015.

Objective: The study was done at a pivotal point in time for both Welch Medical Library and for medical libraries in general. The six physical sites where library services are provided today are a considerable distance from the original vision for the building as a single library service point for the east Baltimore campus. The building provides increasingly inadequate and awkward space for modern library services and staffing levels. At the same time, the rapid shifts from paper-based to electronic library resources call into question how and where future library materials will be stored, and services delivered.

Methods: The plan introduces a network concept that includes a central "hub" and a series of touchdown suites that provide locations for in-person consultations with library staff. This concept extends the "walls" of the virtual library into every aspect of the physical campus, and complements the electronic resources and services available virtually anywhere. The study also incorporates a strategy for adapting the historic Welch Library building in a way that remains consistent with its original mission and emphasizes its importance on the east Baltimore campus. The building will continue to house the Institute of the History of Medicine, expand historical collections, and add the medical archives. The grand study and meeting spaces also original to the building will be restored and expanded, addressing the increasing shortage of such space on campus.

Conclusions: The flexibility and dynamic nature of the Welch plan will support an array of services that can evolve and respond to further changes in library resources and the needs of the Hopkins user community.

INTRODUCTION

Setting

The William H. Welch Medical Library of the Johns Hopkins University is the focal point of the planning and development activities described in this case study. The library is located on the east Baltimore campus of the Johns Hopkins University and provides library services for the faculty, staff, and students of the university's schools of medicine, public health, and nursing, as well as the Johns Hopkins Hospital and affiliated units of the schools and the hospital. The total user population is estimated at 20,000, mostly located on the fifty-two acre campus but also including other Hopkins sites and faculty who travel extensively as a part of their research and clinical practice. Research is a major focus, with research funding totaling over $800 million in fiscal year 2003. The Johns Hopkins Hospital is a large, 1,000-bed, tertiary care facility. Students in the three schools compose approximately 20 percent of the library's user community, and its educational programs emphasize the involvement of students in the research process.

The library has a long tradition of service innovations, including the Welch Library Indexing Project that led to the development of medical subject headings (MeSH), implementation of one of the first integrated library systems, conversion of Victor McKusick's *Mendelian Inheritance in Man* into a searchable online database, and the creation of a research and development unit that is currently taking a lead in educating informatics fellows.[1-2] With an abiding interest in finding the best ways to serve the university's large, research-focused user population, library staff chose to view the challenged state of the physical facilities as an opportunity to conduct a far-reaching architectural study with equal emphasis on service and facilities.

Objective

Although characterized as an architectural plan, the resulting compilation of user feedback, staff input, physical plant assessment, and service evaluation quickly evolved into strategic thinking and a master plan for the future of the Welch Library.[3] It became clear that users sought nontraditional directions for services and delivery methodologies in pursuit of their work. At the same time, Welch librarians explored on-site interactions and expanded their relationships with users outside the physical walls of the library, thereby creating a more integrated approach to the provision of in-person services. This evolution of practice and library science required a unique planning approach to ensure that consistent, user-defined services and resources could be further enhanced and easily obtained without physical dependence on a centrally located facility.

The three-phase architectural plan accomplished these goals by establishing a progressive shift in the idea of library as a place to the more abstract concept of the library as a series of information resources and services. The subtle, yet distinct, difference between the heart pumping and the circulatory system delivering sustenance to the body is one medical model that can be used to describe this variation. The term *convergent architecture,* articulated by Huang, lends itself to the integration of the virtual and physical and to this overall approach of providing rich electronic services as well as in-person services, both of which are highly personalized.[4]

During the first phase described in the plan, touchdown suites will be developed and implemented throughout the campus in key locations, operating in direct partnerships with specific schools and departments. The touchdown suite is a new model in the delivery of library services. Its purpose is to provide convenient services and resources near the place where the user is located and working (see Figure 12.1).

Core services include collaborative information services from a liaison librarian, content-specific electronic resources, customized training classes, tailored technology systems and toolkits, and suite configuration/setup. These touchdown suites are not satellite libraries or the traditional departmental libraries in that they do not contain print material nor is there full-time staffing at the location. The methods section describes the touchdown suites in greater detail.

The second phase of the architectural plan focuses on library operations and staff to better assess the requirements for space to house the important support activities for library resources and services. The Welch Library building constructed in 1929 can no longer adequately support the comprehensive operations required by the library in the twenty-first century. To this end, a new central core facility has been proposed to provide space for library staff. The critical nuance

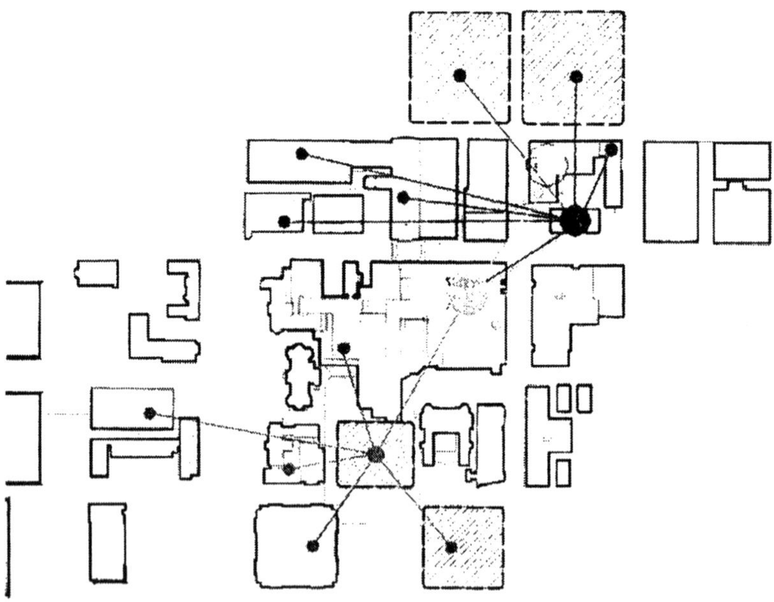

FIGURE 12.1. Distributed library network. Illustration by Will Bryant. Reprinted with permission.

in this shift to a new physical space is that the new facility will not include user space. Instead, it consists only of adequate office space and related functional space for staff needs. Users will be served by the network of touchdown suites throughout the campus and their own direct connections to electronic information resources. This model is predicated on the premise that Welch will no longer manage an on-site physical print collection. In fact, the print collection will be systematically moved to the university's central off-site repository for future electronic retrieval. Because space is no longer needed for users or print collections, the size and location of this new central core facility is not bound by many of the critical space constraints faced by others contemplating new central library facilities.[5]

The final phase of the architectural plan takes into account the historical nature and importance of the Welch Library building on the campus. Although the library's services and resources will no longer emanate from the original building, several other enhanced functions will prosper in the restored physical space. The Institute of the History of Medicine is one of the original cotenants of the Welch building, and its operations will remain in that space. An expanded Historical Library and the addition of the Alan Mason Chesney Medical Archives will colocate two other important information services of the institution. Meeting and seminar space will be created by the restoration of the grand reading rooms, original to the building, thereby addressing in part the increasing shortage of such space on campus.

METHODS

The increasing availability of resource materials in electronic form has increased collaboration between information specialists and the researchers.[6-10] Researchers have responded to this improved access by asking for all needed material to be readily available.[11] The library has moved aggressively in recent years to support both the demand for electronic resources and the related need for more specialized library services. The strategy has been to acquire all the materials it can in electronic form while working to convert older materials into electronic form, and to establish a liaison staff that actively seeks out and assists faculty, staff, and students in their work.

Population Center Touchdown Suite

The Johns Hopkins Population Center (HPC) is one of a number of federally funded centers established to support university-wide research in population sciences, including reproductive health and demography. Recent Welch Library initiatives were noted by HPC associates. In 2003, with a five-year renewal of Center grant funding on the horizon, the director of the HPC approached the library to request that it provide information services to the HPC's research associates and proposed to jointly fund the services with the library.

The former Information Core of the HPC supported its associates by providing a collection of print and electronic materials, document delivery, and expert searching and monthly current awareness services. The existing collection consists of 106 current journal titles, about 6,300 books, and other materials including maps, census data, and the working papers of the Center. One of the Center's most popular services has been the circulation of monthly table of contents to the associates.

In response to this request that the library assume responsibility for information services to HPC associates, the library proposed in July 2003 to develop a touchdown suite, that is, to provide a digital library to researchers working from any location and to offer the new digital library with consultation services from a physical location adjacent to many of the researchers in the Department of Population and Family Health Sciences in the Bloomberg School of Public Health. Toward that end, Welch Library proposed to

- define a collection and services to meet the information needs of the HPC associates guided by an advisory group drawn from among the associates and based on a needs assessment conducted with all associates;
- create the Population Digital Library (PDL) and make it available from any location; identify existing online publications and digitize those that are currently only available in print; and
- offer liaison librarian services to actively seek out and assist researchers, other faculty, and students in their work.

The library also proposed to evaluate the results and share its experience with the HPC, Welch Library advisory committee, and other federally funded population centers. Welch librarians began this work in the fall of 2003. Project team members will plan, implement, test, and report over a two-year period.

Basic Science Research Building (BRB) Touchdown Suite

During the planning phase for a new basic science research building, the library learned that one floor would contain labs, meeting rooms, and a number of shared resources and services of the basic science departments. Recognizing this design as an opportunity to offer on-site support and resources, Welch Library leadership contacted the department chairman responsible for the identified support space. An agreement was reached, and a touchdown space was identified where the basic science liaison librarian could collaborate with faculty, students, and staff, to lead, define, and offer information services. The next section describes the proposed list of services for the touchdown suite in the BRB (see Photo 12.1).

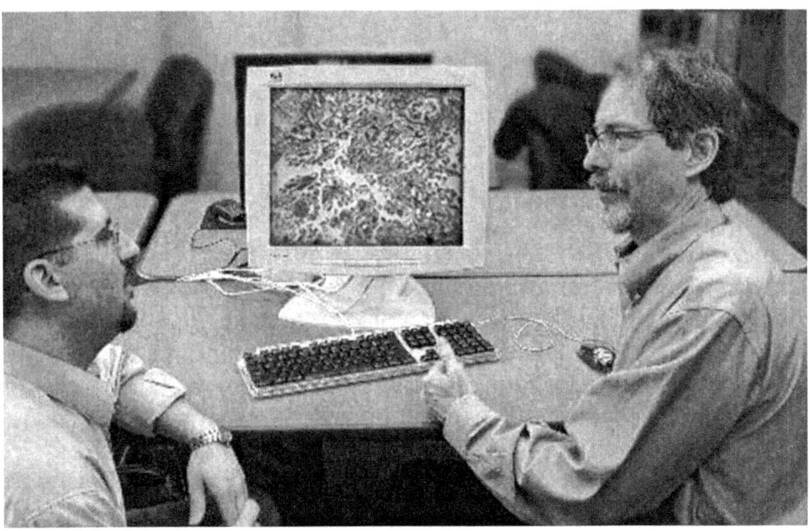

PHOTO 12.1. One-on-one interactive session in the BRB Touchdown Suite. Photo courtesy of Gary Faulkner, Welch Memorial Library. Reprinted with permission.

The basic sciences researchers at Hopkins are affiliated with a number of departments that overlap in many areas of research. For example, yeast research is being conducted in the departments of Molecular Biology and Genetics, Biology, Cell Biology and Anatomy, and Physiology. Basic sciences researchers share many of the same needs regarding resources and services. The outlined services plan was developed to meet such cross-disciplinary information needs in the basic sciences. These services will be explored and tested in collaboration with basic science faculty, staff, and students:

- Customized training courses
- Customized Basic Sciences Research Toolkit Web site
- A partnership between the Library's Advanced Technologies and Information Systems department and the Basic Science Network Office for software hosting
- Office hours for reference and training
- Grant writing and grant application review services and training, assistance with finding funding, and editorial assistance
- Physical space for researchers to use computers
- Ongoing needs assessment

Oncology Training Touchdown Suite

This touchdown suite is different from the others described here, in that it is not as much about a permanent place as it is about a specialized, tailored service. During preliminary touchdown discussions with the education committee at the Sidney Kimmel Comprehensive Cancer Center (SKCCC), oncology faculty members expressed a greater need for training in subject areas as a means of supporting their research activities, than for a place where they could go to meet with a librarian for assistance. The need for training for the administrative staff—the individuals who work in tandem with the faculty on activities such as research paper submission, poster sessions, and reprint file management—was also described as a very high priority for the oncology center.

The library responded with a list of topics that could be offered, based upon the needs and priorities specified by the committee members. The result of a half-year planning effort was a training program titled Academic Productivity Workshop Series: State-of-the-Art Tools and Techniques to Ensure That Your Time and Resources Are Used

Efficiently and Effectively. The program includes a monthly, one-hour lecture offered in a central location at the center.

The library's education program has included instruction on these topics for many years, so preliminary content was readily available.[12] The challenge was to assure that the added specialized content was relevant to both immediate and longer-term needs of the faculty and staff. This goal was accomplished by partnering an education librarian with a faculty liaison from the Center's education committee. The librarian and faculty liaison discussed the content, prepared relevant examples, and jointly reviewed the final presentation prior to the scheduled workshop. Although the specialized content was designed to relate directly to the needs of the oncology center personnel, the lecture topics themselves were also relevant to a much broader audience. The education committee members agreed that publicity should blanket the oncology center, but if others on the campus learned about the existence of the lecture series, they would be welcome to attend. Two strategically placed plasma screens, located in heavily trafficked areas in the cancer research building and the clinical tower, presented the perfect opportunity to announce each lecture. The plasma screens (see Photo 12.2) are used to display information about events scheduled in the oncology center using a PowerPoint slide show. The library created the design and text for each slide announcing a lecture, and education staff at the oncology center assumed responsibility for adding the content to the slide show. Over time, the plasma screens were recognized as the metaphor for the training touchdown center itself. During the current fiscal year, approximately 350 faculty and staff have attended these sessions.

Oncology Patient Information Touchdown Suite

One area identified early in the touchdown suite discussions with the SKCCC was the demand for better methods for meeting patient information needs. Patients' satisfaction with health care is closely tied to the receipt of needed information related to diagnosis and treatment. Oncology health care providers expressed a need for professional assistance in identifying relevant information and structures to provide that information both to clinicians and also directly to the patients.

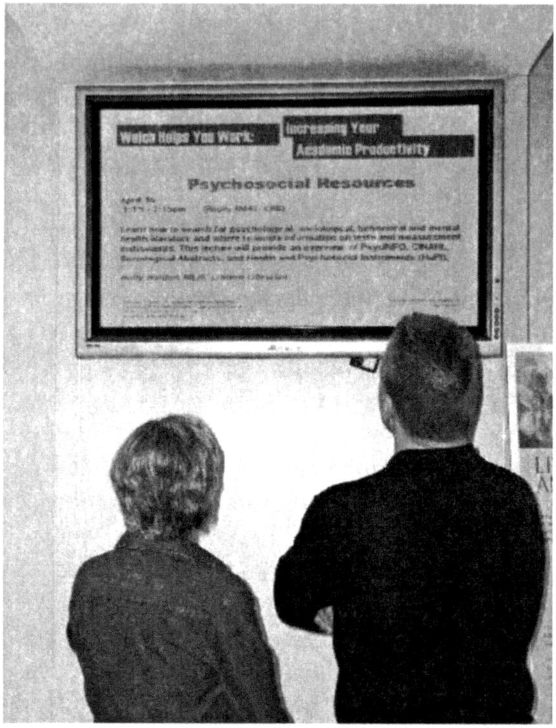

PHOTO 12.2. Faculty and staff view training class announcements on the plasma screen. Photo courtesy of Gary Faulkner, Welch Medical Library. Reprinted with permission.

A team was formed to discuss the patient information needs of the department. The team was composed of a senior oncologist, oncology resident, several oncology nurses whose responsibilities included providing patients with information related to their diagnosis and treatment, and three librarians. The librarians included the liaison program director and two liaison librarians. One liaison librarian serves as liaison to the oncology department, and the other librarian had extensive experience in working with patients to meet their information needs. The discussion was a wide-ranging exploration of current clinical efforts to meet patient information needs and of the range of topics covered by these efforts. The group decided to focus on two areas and develop prototypes to demonstrate the concept of a patient information touchdown. The two prototypes will address brain tumor and colon cancer information. The prototypes are designed to be virtual and adaptable to any physical location at which information is needed. Content areas and types of information for both prototypes have been identified. A beta structure for the brain tumor prototype is available to the project team and is being populated with content.

School of Nursing Touchdown Suite

The library has a long history of managing the Nursing Information Resource Center for the School of Nursing. At the resource center, the faculty and students have access to reference service from full-time staff, computers connected to e-journals, e-databases, and e-reserves, and a modest collection of books and journals. During the spring of 2003, the faculty began to evaluate the resource center to determine if library services, collections (both print and electronic), hours of service, and physical space were actually meeting the needs of the students and were in keeping with the long-term plans for the school. A few faculty members were aware of the library's touchdown initiatives, and were very interested in exploring the feasibility of applying the touchdown model in the nursing school environment.

As a first step, the Dean's office, in collaboration with the library, distributed a comprehensive survey to the nursing school student body to learn more about use of the resource center services, collections, and space. The results of the survey, in addition to circulation reports from the online catalog, showed some interesting trends, some examples of which follow:

- *Print collections:* Nursing students reported infrequent use of print books and journals. Circulation data showed that a large percentage of the collection had circulated fewer than ten times in four years.
- *Study space:* The majority of the students commented that individual study space was very important, but in general, currently available individual study space was adequate. The students also indicated that group study space is extremely important, but that current space for this purpose was woefully inadequate.
- *Computers:* As expected, computer use was very high, and access to e-resources was extremely important. Surprisingly, a

majority of the students reported that the number of computers available for use at the resource center was insufficient to meet study and/or research needs.

- *Course reserves:* Students reported that round-the-clock access to electronic reserves was very important to their research and study needs, but they were disappointed that a small number of courses had reserve material available electronically.
- *Staff:* The respondents stated that they valued the service when it was needed, but the majority reported that library staff was consulted less than once per week.

Library staff and the school discussed this information and how it might be transformed into a realistic action plan, and reached a similar conclusion that this environment was ideal for testing the touchdown model. In order to accomplish this goal within one year, the following actions were recommended:

- Immediately reduce the size of the print collection by eliminating duplicates and titles that had very low circulation.
- Expand the e-reserve library by aggressively increasing the number of course reserves available electronically. During the first year, staff would conduct an active promotion and education campaign to inform the faculty about the benefits for the students and the impact e-reserves would have on their own academic productivity.
- Reduce the reliance need for on-site staff by increasing reliance on electronic or virtual services.
- Create a default home page for the computers in the touchdown suite that would have a joint Welch Library/School logo, and enhance usability by serving as a link to library services such as e-reference, e-reserves, and liaison librarians.
- Expand training opportunities for the faculty and staff using recent experience in oncology as a model.

CENTRAL CORE FACILITY

Planning for library staff space on campus has been actively pursued in numerous building proposals that have recently emerged.

Since, as stated earlier, physical location and adjacencies are not as critical as they were in the past, several opportunities are being explored. The central core space would require approximately 30,000 net square feet, suggesting that library staff be included on one or two floors within a larger building. One important aspect of the planning included a staffing assessment for all library positions to properly project the estimated number of and type of positions that would be required in the future. Another consideration was the close relationship the Welch Library has with the Division of Health Sciences Informatics and the Office of Academic Computing to ensure the continuity of collaborative efforts and expertise sharing.

The Welch Library conducted a department-by-department assessment as part of the architectural study. Library department heads were asked to evaluate future space requirements and staffing needs. Several groups projected significant changes by taking a zero-based approach to this activity in terms of required space needs and the number and level of staff. Formerly large groups such as materials processing, document services, administration, and collection services predicted smaller staffing requirements through anticipated technology advances and shifts from print collection management. In a similar shift, smaller groups such as liaison and outreach activities projected a doubling or tripling of efforts in staffing and resources to meet the anticipated increases in service demand.

In the library's plans for the future, physical infrastructure requirements are also less connected to the facility, but more integrated into point-of-service and mobile technologies. Library staff are no longer required to be "hardwired" to a physical desktop but can opt for less-invasive technology connections. Wireless buildings serving PDAs (personal digital assistants), mobile classrooms, and other transient technologies create workspace and other staff space that are multidimensional and flexible.

One tangible option for the Welch central core facility is a joint-education building being considered by the schools of medicine, public health, and nursing. The location of a central core facility, in support of library services and resources, at the crossroads of education and research activities for the campus is an exciting opportunity.

WELCH LIBRARY BUILDING RENOVATION

The grand restoration of the original Welch Library building is contingent upon the successful completion of phases one and two of the architectural study. The early phases call for a transformation of library-related activities from the overburdened building infrastructure and its original architecture to activities that more suitably fall within the context of the original building, while enhancing its historical role on the campus.

The library building's systems require updating or replacement if they are to continue to adequately support operations of any kind. Eight floors of tiered concrete stacks will no longer be required when the print collection is moved off-site. One of the reading rooms has been converted to staff cubicle offices and public-access computer kiosks. The physical location of the building, toward the northeast corner of the medical campus, is removed from much of the growth that is taking place to the south and west.

Given these limiting factors, the most appropriate mix of occupants and activities for a renovated and repurposed building must be identified. In the future, users will need to be told the difference between the Welch Library and the Welch Library building.

The role of the Institute of the History of Medicine must expand within the renovated building. This long-time tenant has had and will continue to have a prominent presence, an established historical print collection, and faculty responsibilities tied to the history of medicine. The Medical Archives group (currently housed in separate office space) is another potential tenant that would fit well into the restructured building environment.

Many users in the focus groups conveyed the need for various types of meeting space on campus. These included quiet, collaborative spaces for faculty interactions and brainstorming; dining options for faculty, deans, and potential donors; and seminar space for visiting lecturers. One goal is to establish a new Faculty Club within the Welch Library's restored West Reading Room. This reading room once served as the doctors' dining room before it was discontinued due to expanding library operations. Installation of current technology would allow seminars and presentations to be conducted in the new Faculty Club and in the multipurpose meeting space located in the converted stack areas. One or two floors of compact shelving with greater capacity than the existing stack system will provide the required collection storage.

The face-lift for the Welch Library building will not only improve the building infrastructure but will position the facility to serve important and unique cultural and historical needs on campus for many years to come.

CONCLUSION

The three-phased plan articulated in the architectural study is critical to the success of this project. The library must establish successful touchdown suites and build partnerships with users to ensure that their needs are met by this decentralized, yet customized, approach. The work in touchdown suites must evolve into an integrated and seamless collaborative relationship between users and librarians/informationists.[13] The touchdown suites will retain a consistent set of core services to ensure library branding, and allow each suite to be tailored to the individual and varied needs of the user groups.

An active, well-equipped central core facility is essential to provide the necessary infrastructure and support services for the network of touchdown suites and the electronic information resources available throughout the campus. The important behind-the-scenes work by the library support team is critical. The core will also support the continuity of staff and purpose for those remotely located in touchdown suites and for those whose work revolves around the transparent and direct delivery of information resources. Finally, the third phase of the architectural study completes the picture, melding the old and the new, the physical and virtual. The retrofitted library building will be returned to the luster of an earlier time, incorporating new, improved, and modern conveniences in response to reaffirmed needs from the past and emerging needs for the future.

This plan departs from the more traditional thinking of a library as a place in the "heart" of campus life, but it is the best approach for meeting the needs of the research-intensive user community. Pilot touchdown suites are exciting. The library will also gain further experience related to mixing and enhancing physical and virtual services. A new metaphor of the library as the "circulatory system" delivering targeted services and resources wherever needed will carry the Welch Library successfully to 2015 and beyond.

NOTES

1. Koehler, Barbara M., Roderer, Nancy K., and Ruggere, Christine. "A Short History of the William H. Welch Medical Library." *Neurosurgery* 54(February 2004): 465-481.

2. *Informatics Training Program at Johns Hopkins.* Division of Health Sciences Informatics, 2003. Available online at <http://dhsi.med.jhmi.edu/content/training.html>.

3. Rizzo, Joseph and Dugdale, Shirley. *William H. Welch Medical Library Architectural Study.* WelchWeb, 2002. Available online at <http://www.welch.jhu.edu/architecturalstudy/index.html>.

4. Huang, Jeffrey. "Future Space: A New Blueprint for Business Architecture." *Harvard Business Review* 79(April 2001): 149-158.

5. Albanese, Andrew R. "Deserted No More." *Library Journal* 128(April 2003): 34-36.

6. Miller, Ruth H. "Electronic Resources and Academic Libraries, 1980-2000: A Historical Perspective." *Library Trends* 48(spring 2000): 645-670.

7. Okerson, Ann. "Are We There Yet? Online E-Resources Ten Years After." *Library Trends* 48(spring 2000): 671-694.

8. Florance, Valerie, Giuse, Nunzia B., and Ketchell, Deborah S. "Information in Context: Integrating Information Specialists into Practice Settings." *Journal of the Medical Library Association* 90(January 2002): 49-58.

9. Black, Christine, Crest, Sarah, and Volland, Mary. "Building a Successful Information Literacy Infrastructure on the Foundation of Librarian-Faculty Collaboration." *Research Strategies* 18(fall 2001): 215-225.

10. Pearson, David and Rossall, Hannah. "Developing a General Practice Library: A Collaborative Project Between a GP and Librarian." *Health Information and Libraries Journal* 18(December 2001): 192-202.

11. Palmer, Janet P. and Sandler, Mark. "What Do Faculty Want?" *Library Journal Net Connect Supplement* 128(winter 2003): 26-28.

12. *Computers & Communication Classes.* WelchWeb, 2002. Available online at <http://www.welch.jhu.edu/classes/index.cfm>.

13. Florance, Valerie and Davidoff, Frank. "The Informationist: A New Health Profession?" *Annals of Internal Medicine* 132(June 2001): 996-998.

Case Study 13

Library Renovation Planning

Ralph D. Arcari

OVERVIEW

Setting: The Lyman Maynard Stowe Library is the only public academic health center in the geographic area covered by the states of Connecticut, Rhode Island, and western Massachusetts. The library serves the University of Connecticut School of Medicine, School of Dental Medicine, graduate programs in the basic sciences, graduate program in public health, and the John Dempsey Hospital. The citizens of Connecticut are served through Healthnet, the library's consumer health information program. Although the present library opened in April 1973, the building was designed in the 1960s. Consequently, its design was predicated on paper-based information systems that make it ill-suited for accessing electronic library resources and meeting other challenges faced by twenty-first-century libraries.

Objectives: In 2001, a $100,000 contract retained the services of the DuBose Associates architectural firm to plan a library renovation. Objectives included a more user-friendly and welcoming design; multifunctional rooms for study, computer training, and conferences; improved service stations; rest rooms; and an upgraded heating, ventilating, and air-conditioning (HVAC) system to eliminate hot and cold spots and drafts. All planning was limited to the existing 33,000 square feet.

Methods: Architects with DuBose Associates shadowed professional staff as they worked through their daily routines. Focus groups of students and faculty were consulted. A LibQUAL+ survey documented the need for major renovation.

Results: The final plan called for removal of the existing HVAC system, installation of a new duct system, and construction of a new front entrance, single point-of-service desk, twenty-four-hour study room, comfortable reading areas adjacent to the central courtyard, and rest rooms. Construction was substantially completed by February 2005.

Conclusions: Despite the limitations of working with an outmoded design and the confinement of existing space, creative approaches can be used to improve space functionality. The new design will increase on-site library usage as patrons find the new environment more congenial to their research and study needs. Also, the role of professional library staff members as teachers and trainers for e-resources will be facilitated by increased training space in multifunctional rooms, such as the twenty-four-hour study room and other areas.

INTRODUCTION

Background

The library at the University of Connecticut Health Center (UCHC) was named after Lyman Maynard Stowe, the first dean of its School of Medicine. Hired to design UCHC, architect Vincent Kling of Philadelphia envisioned a cathedral to health on a hill in Farmington, about seven miles west of Hartford. The final design was a circular structure with a central courtyard. The library occupies three floors on one side of the courtyard; one floor is below-grade. In 1965, library operations commenced in rented quarters in Hartford, and moved to its present location in April 1973. No renovation work has been done to the library since that date.

UCHC is 1.1 million square feet; the library is 33,000 square feet. Kling apparently saw the library as a reference resource within the context of a large complex. According to his vision, patrons would come to the library to consult printed indexes, photocopy journal articles, and borrow books but return almost immediately to their classrooms, offices, or laboratories. Long-term study would take place in faculty conference rooms or areas set aside in student laboratories. As a result, the Stowe Library lacks rest rooms, closed-door study carrels, and other features. The library does have a positive aesthetic appearance. Twenty-foot windows look out on a courtyard with trees, ivy, and a lawn shaped similar to a Grecian amphitheater.

In the intervening years since its opening, the library has added an audiovisual collection with viewing stations and two computer classrooms, one equipped with PCs, the other with Macs, without any increase in space in the floors above-grade. The below-grade floor, used for journal storage, was expanded in the late 1970s and is now fully occupied with compact storage shelving. The latter provides for collection expansion space estimated to be adequate until 2012.

The centrality of the library's location, immediately inside the UCHC academic entrance and adjacent to classrooms and laboratories on upper floors, is an enduring library asset. However, the Stowe Library's design dates from when libraries functioned as warehouses for paper-based products from publishers. Prior to renovation the library provided extensive e-resources and services despite a crowded, maladapted environment.

Planning Process

In the 2001-2002 academic year, the architectural firm of DuBose Associates, Hartford, Connecticut, was hired to plan a renovation of the Stowe Library. Architects met with library staff, the library advisory committee, and focus groups of faculty and students. In addition, architects shadowed library staff members in each of the library departments.

During this same time period, the library participated in its first LibQUAL+ survey. Survey instruments were sent via e-mail to the UCHC community. Survey recipients were asked to evaluate the library in comparison to their self-perceived standard of expectations. For services and resources, the library met or exceeded expectations. When evaluated as a place, the library was decidedly below expectations.

DuBose Associates operated under two constraints in their renovation planning effort. First, because of the library's location on the inside of a courtyard a build-out was not an option. Second, UCHC administration firmly restricted any renovation to existing library space by declaring that no other space surrounding the library could be affected.

The chorus from students whom the architects interviewed included rest rooms, study rooms that could accommodate up to four individuals, and a twenty-four-hour study room. Many students stated a preference for studying at the newer University of Connecticut Law Library in Hartford's west end. Faculty and library staff believed that an inviting design and more study and computer-based training space were required.

The final plans from DuBose addressed the issues and concerns that library users and staff had brought forward. The front door to the library was to be relocated. The original design has it offset to the side so that patrons make a loop after entering. The space gained by having a central entrance would be used for a twenty-four-hour study room. The original door would stay in place but remain locked during the day. At night, the inside door of the twenty-four-hour study room would be locked and the outside door opened.

A main tenet of the renovation would be a single point-of-service. The reference and circulation desks would be combined and located next to the new entrance (see Figure 13.1). Space savings resulting from this design would be used for rest rooms and a patron services room with stand-up e-mail stations, photocopier, computer printer, and scanner.

An additional tenet was that all rooms be multifunctional so that with wireless laptops they could function as computer classrooms, study rooms, or conference rooms. The computer classrooms would be set up and taken down on an as-needed basis. This latter functionality was particularly important at a time when the information-access training role of the librarian has superseded that of librarian as information retriever. Library design needed to recognize this transition.

Finally, several closed-door study carrels would be added so that patrons could engage in long-term research in the library without having their materials or themselves disturbed. Unfortunately, the architectural review uncovered what library staff members long knew. The heating and ventilation system was so maladroitly designed as to require a completely new system. Discharge and intake air registers were so close together that they caused constant drafts. Temperature sensors were so few in number that a whole zone was cold because a remote sensor was satisfied. Moreover, substantial amounts of asbestos had been used in the ceilings requiring a major asbestos abatement program before any renovation could take place. These considerations would cost over half of the $1.5 million necessary to renovate just the main entrance floor of the library.

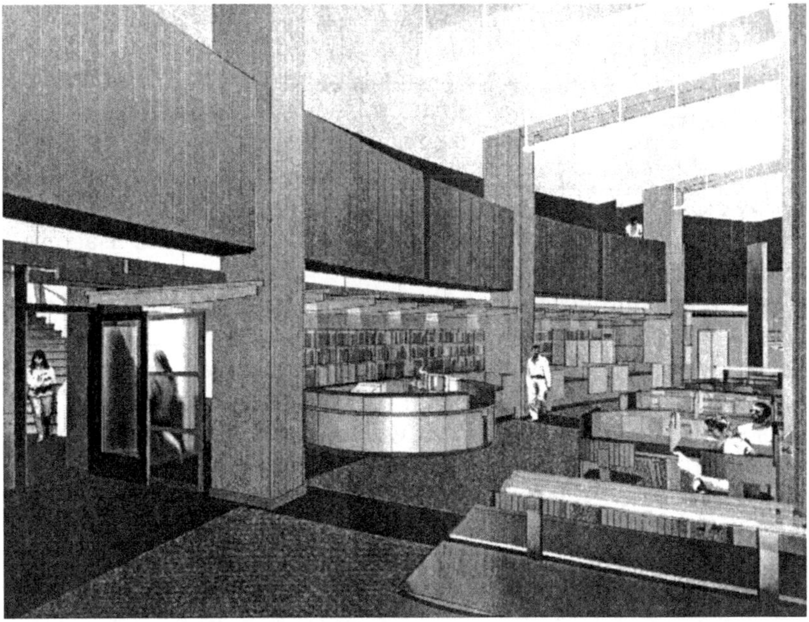

FIGURE 13.1. Architectural rendering of renovated library by Craig Saunders. Reprinted with permission.

The architectural plans prepared by DuBose Associates called for renovation of two floors of the library. Renovations on the second floor included relocation of the History of Medicine room to a more central location to increase its visibility and create a cultural point of interest at the top of the stairway leading from the main to the second floor inside the library. Another major change for the second floor included the multifunctional use of the staff lounge. This area was expanded and equipped with a folding wall. The lounge has a stove, sink, refrigerator, and tables. With the folding door in place, the kitchen area of the lounge could continue to be used and the tables could be equipped with wireless laptops to create a computer-training space. The total cost for the proposed library renovation was set at $2.5 million; $1.5 million for the first floor and $1 million for the second. The renovation Web site is available at <http://library.uchc.edu/ renovation/>.

THE FUTURE

Even though the state of Connecticut agreed to bond itself for $1.3 billion dollars for the ten-year period from 2005 to 2015 for University capital expenditures, it did not appear that the Stowe Library renovation was near the top of the list for this funding. Consequently, efforts were made to make changes that would be consistent with the architects' plans but provide some improvement in space usage and appearance.

All eighty study carrels and chairs have been replaced with new carrels that are wired into the Internet. Access points have been placed in the library for wireless Internet access. A new reference desk was purchased and repositioned for higher visibility (see Photo 13.1). Stacks holding older print indexes were removed from the main floor to the storage area below-grade and easy chairs and couches put in their place. Wireless laptops, stored on a continually recharging cart,

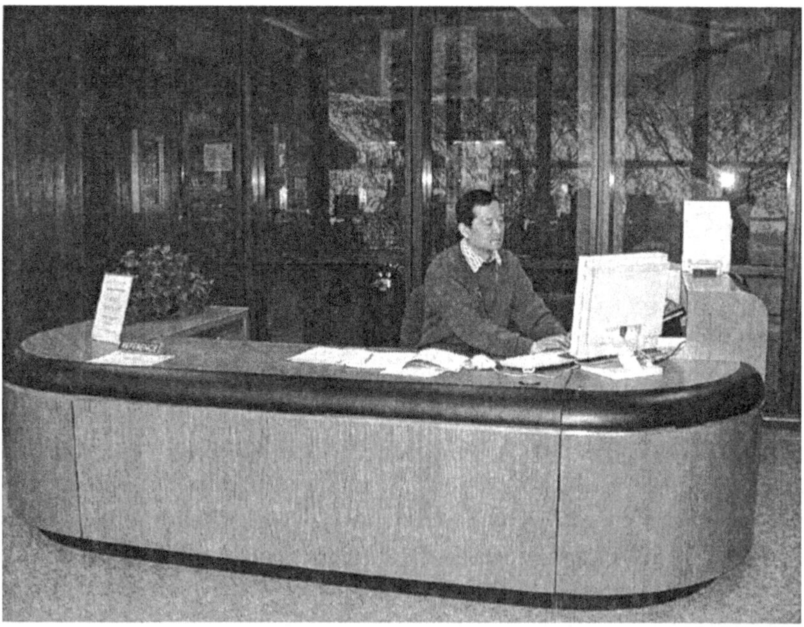

PHOTO 13.1. New reference desk. Photo courtesy of Ralph D. Arcari. Photo by Sheryl Bai. Reprinted with permission.

were acquired so that computer training takes place in existing rooms by setting up the laptops in a classroom configuration and then returning them to their storage cart.

On December 10, 2003, Governor John Rowland held a press conference at the University of Connecticut Health Center to announce his support for $3 million in capital funding to be used for educational expenditures. Of this amount, $1.6 million was earmarked for the Stowe Library renovation. This funding was not part of the ten-year bonding initiative for the university previously noted. With this unexpected funding, much of the proposed architectural planning for the library's main floor was implemented during the 2004 calendar year. Plans included relocating the main entrance door; creating a twenty-four-hour study room; staffing a single point-of-service desk; and installing rest rooms.

Completion of renovation of the library's second floor with funding from the university's ten-year bonding program is not scheduled until fiscal year 2010. The first phase of the renovation started in early April 2004. Contractors have submitted their bids for asbestos abatement and actual construction. Lower bids will result in more funding for furniture, wall coverings, and carpeting.

Library staff weeded the collection in order to reduce the collection as much as possible prior to the start of construction. The reference, monograph, and audiovisual collections were reduced to make more space for study and reading. The latter objective was significant, as use of the library's e-resources is extensive. Annually, there are approximately 750,000 accesses to the library's online catalog, e-journals, e-books, and databases. However, the library gate count has dropped from 250,000 to 185,000 in recent years.

The proposed renovation was designed to help recapture the on-site usage of the library in two ways. First, the creature comforts of the library include soft chairs and couches in open areas near the tall windows to attract users. Second, room multifunctionality allows librarians to more fully exercise their role as teachers and trainers in a time when virtual use of libraries keeps patrons in their offices, laboratories, or classrooms. With more space for training on e-resources and the use of information-technology equipment (e.g., the use of PDAs), more classes and instructional opportunities can be provided through the library.

CONCLUSION

Despite the limitations of working with an outmoded design and the confinement of existing space, creative approaches can be used to improve space functionality. The new design will result in increased on-site library usage as patrons find the new environment more congenial to their research and study needs. Also, the role of professional library staff members as teachers and trainers will be facilitated by increased training space in multifunctional rooms, such as the twenty-four-hour study room and other areas. Renovation of the Lyman Maynard Stowe Library has been a long time in coming. It is anticipated that in 2005 this library will have the look and functionality consistent with a twenty-first-century university by being physically inviting and connected to the Internet in multiple ways. The dedication for the renovated library took place on May 13, 2005.

Index

Page numbers followed by the letter "p" indicate photos; those followed by the letter "t" indicate tables; and those followed by the letter "f" indicate figures.

For Product Safety Concerns and Information please contact our EU representative GPSR@taylorandfrancis.com Taylor & Francis Verlag GmbH, Kaufingerstraße 24, 80331 München, Germany

Batch number: 10725919

Printed by Printforce, the Netherlands